JOURNAL

OF A

STUDENT MIDWIFE

Ellie Ryan

Book Guild Publishing
Sussex, England

First published in Great Britain in 2012 by
The Book Guild Ltd
Pavilion View
19 New Road
Brighton, BN1 1UF

Third printing 2013

Typeset in Garamond by Ellipsis Digital, Glasgow

Printed and bound in Great Britain by
4edge Ltd, Hockley, Essex

A catalogue record for this book is available from
The British Library.

ISBN 978 1 84624 708 8

Dedications

This book is dedicated to my fellow student midwives (you know who you are) . . . It is only because of your constant support and friendship that I got to where I am today. I love you, girls!

A very special thank you goes to my community mentor, who shared her years of midwifery knowledge with me, and whose patience and belief in me allowed my confidence to grow. I would also like to thank all my delivery suite mentors and midwifery lecturers who helped me through, step by step.

A huge thank you to my family; my mum and her partner, my bro and his partner, my little bro, my dad and my father-in-law for their unwavering offers of childcare and constant support through the bad times.

And finally, to my children, I love you both with all my heart. Your smiles, kisses and cuddles make my life complete . . . I have done this all for you.

Contents

Introduction   1

The Interview   9

My Last Months as an Obstetric Theatre and Recovery Nurse   13

My Journey as a Student Midwife   27

Author's Note

For the purposes of protecting anonymity and confidentiality, no names, places or dates have been mentioned at any point through my journal. This ensures that I have abided by the Nursing and Midwifery Council's *Code*.

Introduction

I thought it would be a good idea to keep a reflective journal of my time as a student midwife, so I can look back on the whole experience in years to come. But let's start from the beginning . . . it's been a long journey getting to this point! I first considered midwifery as a career after giving birth to my daughter. HUGE cliché, I realise that now, but for me it was 100% true and it was at this time that becoming a midwife became my ambition. I wanted to be able to give to other women the precious gifts that my midwives had given me; to feel special, cared for, have all those niggling questions answered (no matter how silly I felt they might be), to feel supported, empowered and in control of what was happening. I didn't want to do this straightaway – I wanted to enjoy my own baby and my husband and I knew we wanted another baby to complete our family before long.

A year and a half later I fell pregnant again, but this time I had an active eighteen-month old to look after too! During my pregnancy, I struggled through a time of huge uncertainty. My GP rang me one day and asked how I was; my response was to think the worst and I broke down on the phone. He explained that the results of my blood test (the triple test) confirmed a one in eighty risk of my baby having Down's Syndrome and that I needed to have an amniocentesis. I was only twenty-two years old, and had naively thought that this only happened to women in their forties. He arranged for the hospital to ring me straightaway with my appointment details (it was the next day), and my community midwife arrived within half an hour. Bless her; she sat patiently whilst I sobbed my heart out. The following day I had the amniocentesis, refusing all pictures of my baby, although when I got home I found the sonographer had popped some into the back of my handheld notes for me. I then had to wait for three weeks for the test results. During the wait, I began to feel my baby moving. I felt awful. I wanted to be happy . . . I could feel my baby inside me but it was as if a blanket of sadness had been wrapped round me. I cried a lot during those weeks. Then came the day of the results. The phone rang; it was a lady from the hospital with an overly-kind tone of voice. She asked some questions to confirm it was me she was speaking to and then she told me my baby was healthy. I cried again, but this time tears of happiness! She asked me if I wanted to know the sex of my baby. I knew this was coming; they had explained this to me before, the test looked at the baby's genes and from that they obviously knew the sex. My husband and I had decided that after what we had been through, we wanted to know. I was having a boy! My husband cried when I phoned him. It was the perfect ending to our little drama, a healthy baby boy. He was born – or rather flew into the world after just three big pushes – the following March.

During the years when my children were babies or toddlers, I chose to continue working part-time in a call centre so I was able to be at home as much as possible for my children, and see them growing up. But all the time in the back of my mind, a plan was forming; when they were both in school, I would begin my training.

When my son was a couple of years old I started researching midwifery and contacted local colleges and universities. What I hadn't banked on was the popularity of the midwifery course. Perhaps all women who had had babies dreamt of becoming midwives . . . it certainly seemed that way!

By chance, I saw a job advertised at my local hospital. It was as an Accident and Emergency (A&E) twilight receptionist (working from 9p.m. to midnight 3 or 4 days a week). I thought about applying; it would mean I could continue part-time in the call centre, and by 9p.m. my little ones were safely tucked up in bed, so it wouldn't affect my time with them. It would also give me an introduction into working in a hospital environment with nurses, other medical staff and patients, so I applied and got the job. Actually, I loved working in a hospital and the busyness of working in A&E – it was brilliant! I was only booking patients in, getting their notes and sorting out paperwork, but I was part of the team. I found I could relate to patients, I could talk to them easily and made lots of cups of tea! My path even crossed that of the midwives on a couple of occasions. One poor woman didn't make it up to the delivery suite and had her baby in the car outside A&E. I had to push another woman in a wheelchair at full speed up to the delivery suite. Luckily we made it in time! But there were sad times too. There had been an awful car accident one evening and I got to work to find a baby's car seat in my reception area. It was covered in blood. Both mum and baby were in the resuscitation room. Mum survived the accident, but baby didn't. Seeing a woman in such emotional turmoil was horrendous. How on earth can you comfort someone in that position? The nurses were amazing. I tried to stay out of the way, but we all cried together at the end of that shift.

A few months later I saw a poster on one of the hospital notice boards; there was going to be a midwifery open evening. I went along and was surprised at how many other women were there, all as eager as me to become midwives. We sat and listened to the midwifery lecturers explaining the course, the commitment required, the practical placements, the academic work and – shock horror – exams. I hadn't done those since flunking my A-Levels when I was seventeen! At the end of the evening, the midwife who had been speaking came over to me (to the envy of the other women). She said she just had to come and speak to me because I looked so familiar. I couldn't place her, although in the car on the way home it suddenly hit me. After delivering my son, my midwife had to call for assistance from the senior midwife because my placenta was taking its time to come out. This involved supporting me whilst I crouched on the bed and peed into a bedpan, and then gently pulling the umbilical cord to ease the placenta out. It was her; she had been the senior midwife on duty that day!

Fortunately, I hadn't remembered that when she approached me and I chatted away to her happily. I explained my reasons for wanting to become a midwife, and asked her about the entry requirements for the course. Hooray! Five GCSEs, grades 'A'–'C', including Maths and

English. I had those! Fantastic! But that was for the diploma, and they wanted all students to do the degree. Ouch that hurt... hopes up so high and then bang... back down to earth with a bump. Quickly recovering, I went on to find out that at least two A-Levels were required and evidence of recent academic study. Why oh why didn't I study for my A-Levels when I had the chance? Oh yeah, I remember, my social life was far more important at the time! Should have listened to my parents. The senior midwife encouraged me to contact the local regional college to find out about A-Level evening courses and an access to nursing course, which would also be acceptable.

Big dilemma . . . what was I going to do? The thought of having to take two A-Levels felt like suddenly having a brick wall in front of me; they would have nothing to do with midwifery. Could I manage it? Would I stay motivated? The access course was full-time for two years or part-time for a million years! A girly night in with my best mate (a nurse) and a bottle of red was needed. We chatted and drank . . . our words became slurred but it came to me, in a moment of clarity! I would train as a nurse (it would be an introduction to the healthcare profession) and then do this midwifery conversion course my mate was telling me about. I could do it! Maybe that was the red wine talking, but over the next few weeks I knew that this was going to be my future.

I enrolled for an A-Level Sociology evening class (evidence of recent study) and put my application in for the adult nursing course (I had the GCSEs required) which would be starting the following September. Whilst I was waiting to hear if I had been invited for an interview for the nursing course, I was hard at work with my sociology studies. I surprised myself; it was good fun! And I could do it! Life at home continued as normal with my daughter at school and my son at playgroup. Then the bombshell; I was being made redundant. The call centre I was working in was closing and the work moving to India. It would happen within nine months. Everything now depended on getting onto the nursing course.

To cut a very long story short, I was offered a place on the nursing course. The redundancy money from the call centre helped to top up my bursary and I left my twilight job in A&E. For the next three years I was a student nurse . . . how I wish I had kept a journal of that experience! There were highs and lows, sad times and happy times, times I knew I could do it and times I wanted to quit. Times when all I could think about was becoming a midwife. I gradually found out that most of my fellow student nurses had exactly the same idea as me; qualify as a nurse and then do midwifery. Would I ever actually be a midwife? Being a student nurse did give me the opportunity to spend time with midwives; two days to be precise. The first day was spent in an antenatal clinic. Fantastic . . . it was all worth it after all . . . I was learning how to palpate women's abdomens to feel the position of the baby. This was more like it! I soaked up all the information I was given and thoroughly enjoyed my day in clinic. The second day was spent making home visits to new mums and their newborn babies. Wow . . . I was introduced to the process of postnatal mum and baby checks, but the thing I most enjoyed was sitting and talking to these women and their partners about their experiences. It refreshed my motivation; I was going to do this!

As a student nurse I had a four-week elective placement that involved me arranging my own work experience, something I was interested in and hadn't yet done. What else could I do but try and get a placement on the delivery suite and postnatal ward? Whether it was pure luck or perseverance I don't know, but I got it . . . Four whole weeks working with midwives on the delivery suite and postnatal ward. What an opportunity! The postnatal ward was first; I completely immersed myself in my work, and with the support of a couple of amazing midwives, felt myself going from strength to strength. I was being introduced to midwifery terminology, and learning how to relate to women and their babies. It wasn't all a bed of roses; this was the NHS after all. Staff shortages, budget freezes and all these women having babies meant it was hard work. Hard work, but wonderful!

Then came my two weeks on the delivery suite; would I be able to cope with observing a baby being born? What if, after all this time and effort spent on trying to realise my dream, I hated it? I was panic-stricken . . . all my confidence disappeared. I was looking forward to it, it was what I wanted, but I was so nervous. What was it going to be like? My mentor had been a nurse, and then trained as a midwife. She was fab, easy to talk to and respectful of my own ambitions. I had the most amazing two weeks with her. The first labouring woman we cared for scared the living daylights out of me. The pain of the contractions consumed her, my communication skills (which previously I thought were top-notch) crumbled and all I could do was step back and watch my mentor support her through her labour. I did a couple of blood pressures, took her pulse, fetched a few cups of water and uttered the odd 'You're doing brilliantly' and 'Fantastic push!' Then WOW! Her baby girl was born. This new baby was here! Mum was crying, Dad was crying, Baby was crying and yes, you guessed it, I was crying too. Incredible! I felt so honoured to have been there. What a privilege to see this beautiful little girl being born! The rest of my time on delivery was a whirlwind of learning experiences. I saw vaginal and Caesarean deliveries, and my first shoulder dystocia, which is where the baby's head delivers but the shoulders get stuck, a true obstetric emergency that can cause the death of the baby (terrifying), and I was in awe of how calm and reassuring the midwives were when working under such pressure. I came away feeling more determined than ever.

I qualified as a nurse. Brilliant timing . . . the NHS was in turmoil and jobs were scarce. The rotation job I had managed to bag was suddenly gone due to lack of funds, although I was given a month's pay in compensation. I applied for everything going; three jobs, but there was just one I really wanted. It was as an obstetric theatre and recovery nurse. Competition for jobs was fierce; I felt I had no chance, but applied anyway, hoping and praying. What happened that month was, well, completely bonkers! The three interviews I had been invited for went well, and I was offered all three jobs. There were no agonising hours spent deliberating over which job to take. I knew which one I wanted. And so, six weeks later, after a sleepless night I got out of bed at 5.30a.m. and began my journey to work as an obstetric theatre and recovery nurse!

Could life be any better than this? Here I was, working as a nurse on a delivery suite! How lucky was I? The transition from student nurse to qualified nurse was terrifying. We had been warned by our lecturers at university that the experience was going to be difficult, but all of a sudden I was accountable for providing nursing care to patients who had just had major surgery (Caesarean sections) and who had newborn babies. Words can't describe the panic I felt each time a woman's blood pressure wasn't normal, or when I found protein in a urine sample . . . Thankfully, I was well supported, and not left to my own devices, unlike some of the girls who had qualified with me and who were having an awful time of it on the wards. I had the enormous task of learning how to be a scrub nurse in front of me. All of those instruments . . . how on earth was I ever going to remember what they were all called, let alone what they were all for? It happened gradually, although quicker than I initially thought. I was doing it! Scrubbing for C-sections, not panicking, watching new life being brought into the world each and every day. And I continued to care for women and their newborn babies in the recovery room. Three years of hard work had paid off. I got up in the morning looking forward to going into work. I loved my job. It was the best job in the world! Maybe I would do this for a while, and then go on to midwifery in a couple of years. Then one day I was at home, knackered from the incredibly busy shift I had had the day before (seven C-sections, short of staff, no breaks – the usual) and the phone rang. It was my tutor from uni. Odd. Why was she ringing me? Had there been a mistake? Was I not a qualified nurse after all? She knew about my longing to be a midwife, we had talked about it on many occasions (she was a nurse and a midwife herself). She wanted to make sure I knew that the next midwifery conversion programme that the uni was running was going to be the last. The last? That couldn't be right; I loved my job and I wanted to stay there, for a little while at least . . . If I couldn't do the conversion in a couple of years what was I going to do? She explained that the three-year direct entry midwifery programme was being pushed as the only option. If I wanted to do the shortened eighteen-month conversion I had to apply now. What was the point in thinking this one through? I knew what I had to do, and I applied that day. Within a few weeks the letter arrived. This was it, the moment of truth. Had my application got through the first round of sorting? Had I been offered an interview? I couldn't open it. That evening we sat down for our tea together (I needed my kids' and hubby's support!!). I showed them the unopened letter, which resulted in the usual argument between the kids about who would open it. My husband opened it in the end; with a poker face he read it and put it down. I couldn't read him and was MAD! How could he tease me over something this important? I was just about to let vent my frustration when he smiled. I had an interview, the following week! Oh my God, only a week to prepare. Was I working? I couldn't tell them at work; no I was off, relief! The kids were jumping around the table chanting 'Mummy's gonna be a midwife!' They were both so sweet. I had to try and explain to them (they were still only nine and seven years old) that I had to be fantastic at the interview and be offered a place . . . it was by no means guaranteed.

The Interview

The day of the interview arrived. How could I keep putting myself through this? I was too nervous to sleep the night before. I had dreamt about losing a baby at work and finding it in the sluice after a frantic search! Bizarre. I got there, an hour early. I needed a cigarette (I promised myself I would stop if I got on the course; was unhealthy and smelt yucky!), so parked at the deserted end of the car park in front of a bush, and wound the window down. All too quickly it was time to go inside, so I popped a couple of mints in my mouth and had a quick squirt of perfume. My hands were shaking. I picked up my portfolio, and all the proof of identity I had been told to bring with me for the Criminal Records Bureau check. I could hardly walk straight. Pull yourself together; you've made it this far. Into the building, across to the reception, signed in... loo, where's the loo? The receptionist pointed to it with a smile on her face. I dashed for the loo and peed for England! Back out to reception, over to the seats, four other women there already . . . this was who I was up against! After fifteen minutes a lady walked across to us, introduced herself as a midwifery lecturer and asked us to follow her.

We sat down in a classroom. There were six of us now, and she asked us to introduce ourselves to the group. Yuk! Hate doing this, my cheeks always glow red! All the others had been nursing for years. There was no hope, why would I get chosen? After listening to an outline of the course we were asked to fill in a skills sheet. This was it. Was definitely not going to get through this bit . . . what was the calculation for IV drugs again? Flow rates, flow rates . . . how did you work them out? Did it every day at work, but . . . oh, my mind's gone blank. I had the piece of paper in front of me. Could I look at it?

Was there any point? What the heck, am here now, might as well try. Relief, a wave of relief was flooding over me. All I had to do was tick what clinical skills I regularly used. No hard maths calculations! I ticked it all, apart from venepuncture; I still needed to do the Trust study day before I was able to do that. Not so bad after all!

Then I heard the thing I had been dreading. 'We have a little surprise task for you,' said the interviewer. What could it be? Role play, I bet it's role play, I hate role play. 'We have a short written exercise for you to complete, it should take about forty-five minutes.' An essay, this would be OK, I like writing essays, am good at that. This isn't so bad! We all looked at each other, the others looked panicked. I tried to give a reassuring (but not smug) smile. You have two titles to choose from; answer whichever you feel more confident with. Two choices – even better – must be able to do justice to one of them! Here we go, what do they want us to write about? OK, so I had the choice of 'Why do you want to become a midwife?' and 'What qualities does a person need to become an effective midwife?' Well, I had already written about why I wanted to become a midwife on my application form, so what was the point in answering that again. So I answered the second one. We sat in silence; the interviewer had left us to it. This was OK, just had to keep it together for a bit longer. Buzz, buzz, buzz . . . oh no, that was my phone in my bag. Someone had sent me a text message. Should I get my phone out? Didn't want the others to think I was cheating in some way. It went off again. I had to get it out and turn it off. Back to the essay, only ten minutes left and I still had so many ideas in my head to get down on paper. Finished. Done.

We were told it was the individual interviews next: 'You can decide between yourselves which order you would like to come in.' Me first, me first, get it over and done with! No, hang on, maybe this is some sort of groupwork task. Nobody was speaking so I broke the ice and said something about fighting it out between ourselves. Went down like a lead balloon. So I volunteered the information that I didn't mind when I went in, if the others had childcare or work commitments (it was my day off and the kids were at school). Then everyone said they had to get back to their kids. Am I manipulative or what?

They have all just openly stated how inflexible they can be. No, that's too mean; I am not manipulative, I was just trying to negotiate the best for everyone. The result: I am last to be interviewed. Great.

I waited for my turn. Was so nervous, don't really remember what I chatted about with the other girls also waiting. The first girl came out, she didn't look happy. She just went on and on about how badly it went and how she'd blown it. We tried to be supportive. It couldn't have been that bad, surely? About two hours later I was on my own. The others had gone, and I was waiting to be called in. This was it. I walked in, shook hands, sat down and was offered a glass of water. What happened next is still a blur. I explained why I wanted to be a midwife; that my motivation was to support women through their pregnancies, births and the initial postnatal period and why I had done my nursing first. I talked about my elective placement with the midwives and how I felt the challenge of the midwifery course was going to be studying at degree level, as I'd only studied at diploma level in the past. I talked about my kids and the support I had from my husband, about being a student and finally I talked about my job as an obstetric theatre and recovery nurse (this seemed to impress them if nothing else did). I do remember them asking me over and over again in different ways why I wanted to be a midwife. I kept thinking I'd explained that already, and I began questioning whether I was actually answering the question, or whether I was rabbiting on and getting myself sidetracked. The ordeal was finally over and I was told I would have a letter by the following Thursday; they still had fourteen more to interview. That would be twenty in total that I knew about, and only five places were being funded. Had I done enough to get through?

That weekend I was like a bear with a sore head. I tried not to snap at the kids and hubby . . . I tried to keep busy. Back at work I wanted to tell them all. But how could I? I had only been there a month or so and had already applied for something else. They were all so kind, teaching me my new job and helping me, making me feel part of the team. Finally it was Thursday, which also happened to be my graduation day. We had to be out of the house early, before the post had arrived. I felt the usual pangs of envy when the midwives were up on stage receiving their diplomas and degrees. Could have been me . . . still might be. At last, I am on the way home, I can see letters through the front door. Grab them. Nothing. This went on for another week. Should I ring the uni? No. Don't want to appear desperate or pushy. Patience is a virtue.

Ten days later, I had just come back from dropping the kids at school and was feeling very sorry for myself. I felt useless and low, like it had all been a waste of time. I opened the front door and there it was. THE letter. I don't know what came over me, but I dropped my bag, grabbed the letter and ripped it open. Thank you for attending for interview, we hope you enjoyed your visit, yeah, yeah, yeah . . . get to the important bit . . . I am pleased to be able to offer you a place on the midwifery programme. At this point I shrieked at the top of my voice and started dancing round the kitchen. My poor dog didn't have a clue what was going on and was barking and jumping around the kitchen too! YES! I HAVE DONE IT! This is what I have worked so hard for and it is finally going to happen!

My last months as an Obstetric Theatre and Recovery Nurse

Twenty-six weeks to go . . .

Monday

This is it, the year that I will become a student midwife! I am so excited – words cannot describe it!! Only six months to wait before my course starts. I had the new Next catalogue delivered the other day and have ordered a whole new wardrobe for when I start as a student midwife. When I start as a student midwife . . . still hasn't really sunk in! I have told a couple of close friends at work, and have sworn them to secrecy. What with this new Agenda for Change initiative I now have to give two months' notice, so have planned to make it general knowledge when I hand in my resignation. That way I will finish and I can spend a couple of weeks at home with the kids (although they will be at school). It will be nice to have those weeks of normality before the whirlwind of being a student begins again. At least this time I will continue to be paid and not have to manage on a bursary!

Thursday

Clothes I ordered arrived. Definitely make me look like a midwife! Found a fab website too, Student Midwives Sanctuary. Have got some advice on the books I need to get from it. Just counting down the days now. Was at work the other day doing statutory training (with the midwives) and one of the midwifery lecturers from uni came and gave us a little talk. She confirmed that the last eighteen-month conversion programme was starting in the summer and all five students had been chosen. I wanted to get up and shout 'It's me, it's me . . . I have been chosen!' but thought better of it. Especially seeing as my manager was in the room. But I did find out that the course starts on my birthday. That's fate; it was meant to be!

Twenty-five weeks to go . . .

Thursday

Have just finished reading *Baby Catcher* by Peggy Vincent. Couldn't put it down. Read it in a day and a half! It was truly inspirational. I laughed out loud, I cried, and experienced a true roller coaster of emotions. Am sure my fellow shoppers in Tesco this morning thought I was a loon, walking around chuckling to myself as I had flashbacks of some of the more quirky bits of the book (the goose especially!). What a book – a must-read for student midwives everywhere.

Twenty-three weeks to go . . .

Friday

Worked yesterday with a lovely healthcare assistant (HCA) who had an interview for the direct entry midwifery course a couple of days ago. She was really depressed, bless her. The interview had gone well, but with only eight places available and another three months of interviews taking place, she doesn't feel as if she has a chance. She has a degree (and student loan) already, and got her job in the obstetric theatres to expand her experience of working within midwifery, but was told that the bursaries were no longer available. Then at lunchtime we were all sitting in the midwifery staff room and a couple of the HCAs from the delivery suite were saying they also have interviews for the same course next week. There are so many women out there who want to become midwives, I realise that not everyone can train – there would be thousands of surplus midwives! But it really is a struggle to even get an interview, let alone be offered a place . . . I feel so thankful that I have got this far.

Nineteen weeks to go . . .

Monday

Have had a week off and am back tonight for a run of three nights. Am working with another nurse tonight but for nights two and three will be on my own for the first time, with just an HCA for support. Have never ever been so frightened! I know I am a nurse, but have only been for a few months, and anything could come round the corner from the delivery suite. Just keep repeating 'Please let all births be vaginal on Tuesday and Wednesday night, please let all births be vaginal on Tuesday and Wednesday night . . .'

Thursday

Oh my God. I am knackered. Have survived my nights, but only just! My first night alone, I had a woman whose haemoglobin dropped to half the normal level and subsequently needed three units of blood; an emergency section for PET (pre-eclampsia); a placental abruption (placenta haemorrhages before baby is delivered, which is life-threatening to mother and baby) where the baby was born with undiagnosed Down's syndrome, and another emergency section for failure to progress in labour. Baptism of fire or what! Then last night, I thought it couldn't get any worse, and it did! Got to work and they were just taking a trial (trial of instrumental delivery, if it fails it becomes a section) into theatre, then we got a fourth degree tear repair, then an emergency section followed very quickly by a crash section in which the baby was delivered looking white and floppy which was scary (baby was OK), then an ARM (artificial rupture of membranes) done in theatre because the baby's head was high and the doctors were worried it may be a possible cord prolapse, and finally just as the morning girls were coming on, another emergency section was brought round . . . and breathe! Managed to drink half a cup of tea, and didn't get to sit down all night. I did it though, all by myself. Bring it on!

Nine weeks to go . . .

Monday

Am still counting down the days to becoming a student midwife! Seems like it's going so slowly, but so quickly at the same time . . . weird! Lots has happened. I have now handed my notice in. I had originally decided to have at least a couple of weeks off before starting my midwifery, but my manager persuaded me to stay, so I will go from one to the other with a weekend to get my head together! It has been a real mix of emotions, which I wasn't expecting at all. I love my job, and will be very sad to leave, but I know that I will be going on to do something I have always wanted to do. I suppose the thought that keeps coming back to me is that maybe I won't manage, academically or when out on placement. The thought of failing is awful. Everyone has been really encouraging; my manager has been fab, as have all my colleagues and family too. Just can't help thinking that I am giving up this amazing job. I suppose it's only natural to feel nervous and anxious when you have made a decision that will affect your life in such a big way. Don't get me wrong; midwifery is what I have worked towards for years and now I am nearly there I can't believe I feel so panicky! I just wish I could get hold of the admissions tutor at uni. Now I have handed my notice in, it would be good to have some written confirmation of the exact start date, get my contract, and know if/when I have any summer leave! The university did ring me a few weeks ago to confirm I had been given occupational health clearance to start, so at least that's one hurdle done and dusted. From talking to the girls at work who have applied for the direct entry midwifery programme, I know that the admissions tutor is going to have her hands full at the moment, with lots of people wanting to speak to her, so I guess I will just keep trying!

Enough of the whingeing. Work has been fabulous, from a learning perspective. Have come across quite a few things I haven't been involved with before including placenta accreta (woman bled a lot and needed lots of blood transfused during C-section!); triplets; more twins; a grunting baby (which needed help with breathing) and a baby born with spina bifida. Then there are the things which are just part and parcel of the job, but which are so rewarding, like helping new mums latch babies to their breast to start feeding, reassuring them and seeing these women bonding with their babies.

Oh, almost forgot, have invested in a few more books for my midwifery library. One is a midwifery handbook, looks like it has just about everything in it! One is about breastfeeding and is packed with lots of advice, so must have a good read. The other is a book called *Call the Midwife* by Jennifer Worth and is her memoirs of being a midwife in London during the 1950s. Can't wait to read it! Am on nights again this week, so maybe I will get the chance to start it, although I do want to re-read the Harry Potter books before the next film is out! Priorities . . . ha ha ha . . .

Eight weeks to go . . .

Wednesday

Finally, the letter I have been waiting for has arrived! Confirmation that the midwifery conversion course starts on my birthday at 9a.m. I have to get three passport-size photos and complete all the forms (including a uniform request form) and send them back as soon as possible with a cheque for £60 (uni registration fee). I also have the timetable for the next eighteen months and although it's very basic, I can see that my first stint on the delivery suite will be three months after I start, but before that I get six weeks in the community, which will be fantastic! Will have to wait three months before I get a week's leave though, which is a shame; was hoping to have at least one week off whilst the children are on their summer holidays. Am off to have a shower and wash my hair so I look at least semi-human in my passport photos.

Friday

Was allocated to be scrub nurse in theatre today, which I love. The first woman, having an elective Caesarean, was being looked after by a student midwife who is just about to finish the conversion programme. I managed to get ten minutes with her at lunchtime, and she has scared me BIG time! She was very positive about the course, and said she has loved every minute of it, but she said it takes over your life. She described the last eighteen months as living, breathing, eating and sleeping midwifery! The academic side sounds quite full-on too. Not that that particularly worries me, I do like writing essays, but it goes back to the same anxieties . . . Will I cope?

Our elective section list was only for the morning and we were there just to deal with emergencies for the afternoon. Surprisingly we were having a quiet day. Should never say that . . . have learnt this by now. All of a sudden we had twins on the way round for an emergency section because of an unreassuring CTG (cardiotocography), and delivery suite had a phone call from a community midwife who was dealing with an undiagnosed breech at a planned home birth and they were on their way. We were on standby to do an emergency section, but she delivered in the ambulance en route, so our services in theatre weren't required after all. These babies! Some of them do make a dramatic entrance into the world!

Five weeks to go . . .

Friday

Contract arrived in the post this morning. Only problem is it's for the wrong NHS Trust. The university I am going to covers quite a few Trusts, so spent half the morning on the phone trying to sort it all out. Have managed to, with the help of the lead professional midwife at the Trust I was originally told I was going to, and still am going to (thankfully, because it's only ten minutes from where I live). So yet another mini-drama over, and I can look forward to the next four weeks of being a nurse.

One of the midwives who qualified recently has sold me all her midwifery books. Was so thrilled she thought of me. So my little midwifery collection has become a huge collection. Will have to try and make space on my bookcase – think it's about time I put all my nursing lecture notes in the attic!

Four weeks to go . . .

Thursday

Have just woken up after finishing my last-ever week of nights in theatres. It was a good set of nights; managed everything and not too busy. Hate the drive home at the end of a shift though. Never mind, it's done now and only three weeks left till I start . . . can't quite believe it! Am trying to hide my excitement when I am at work because one of the HCAs (who has now become a very good friend) has found out that she has not got a place on the direct entry midwifery programme at the same uni I will be going to. She had her interview a few months ago, and has been waiting all this time to find out. She would be a fantastic midwife, and I can't believe that they have said 'no' to her. She's devastated. It's all she has wanted to do for the last few years and this is her second year of applying. She now says that she isn't going to bother applying again, ever. She is going to go abroad and travel, but I really hope she does re-apply, at some point in the future. I think she is emotionally worn out and just needs time to get her head back together. I know she is dedicated to becoming a midwife, just hope she gets the opportunity.

Three weeks to go . . .

Thursday

The midwife from the hospital I will be based at called me today. She has finally received all my paperwork from the uni and was just checking what band I am on for wages. She reassured me that my contract is being put together now and I will have it shortly. I checked my emails after lunch and she had sent me a copy of an email she had sent to another midwife about me. It was about sorting out which community team I was going to be allocated to, and arranging an induction/orientation package for me. She has been so helpful. I replied to thank her, and to say how much I appreciated her help and how I was really looking forward to joining her team and the amazing experiences I had ahead of me. The uni had been useless, so having someone who seemed to actually care about me was fantastic! Within an hour she emailed me again, saying she was glad to be of help. She also confirmed that they operate a self-rostering system for student midwives at the hospital, they have found this works very well and is very flexible! Couldn't ask for anything more than this really, knowing that I will be able to self-roster when on delivery suite and the postnatal ward is such a relief. It will make things so much easier for me, and will allow me a little flexibility, so hopefully I will still manage a lot of time with my children.

Two weeks to go . . .

Monday

Two weeks today and I will be a student midwife at uni, being given all my paperwork . . . maybe having my first lecture. Am starting to get butterflies when I think about it!

Bought a new A4 pad of lined paper ready for taking notes; it has a pink cover, nice and bright! After taking the kids to school this morning I came home and prepared my pencil case . . . black, blue and red pens . . . pencil . . . ruler . . . calculator . . . highlighter pens. Need to get a little notebook small enough to pop into my pocket so I can jot down things as I come across them when I am on placement. I found this really handy as a student nurse, because at the end of a shift I would get home and look up all the things I had written down and learn about them. Also compiled a wish list of midwifery books

I would like, and have emailed it to all my family ready for my birthday in two weeks' time. Am a cheeky moo I know, but what the hell!

Only six more shifts left at work. It's starting to hit me now, I won't be there for much longer at all. Because they operate a long day-shift system, I am already working shifts for the last time with various people. It's so sad. We have arranged a leaving do on Friday, just a meal and then bowling, so it will be nice to see everyone outside of work. I hate goodbyes though, and am not good at them at all.

Friday

So far this week I have worked Wednesday and Thursday. I had a lovely pampering day with my mum on Tuesday, but work were short of staff so I agreed to work today too (will also be working tomorrow). So, will have done four in a row by the end of the week – must be mad! Today was horrendous. Arrived at work to find myself taking handover for a very poorly patient in recovery. After half an hour or so had to call medical staff because her Hb had dropped very low and she was symptomatic. Took all morning to stabilise her for transfer to the ward. Whilst I was busy with this, the three elective sections were taking place one after the other, so recovery was filling up too. I had just discharged my lady to the ward when an emergency section came round. I was sent to scrub for this one. Baby was delivered, and was very flat. Paediatricians were there, but the Resuscitaire wasn't working properly so they had to run with the baby into another theatre. The baby was OK but needed to go to NICU (neonatal intensive care unit). Then we did another three emergencies and twins. I was working a bank shift till 3p.m. so left (feeling very guilty).

I arrived back at work at 7.30p.m. to meet the girls for my leaving do, and, bless them, they all looked knackered. It had carried on like that all afternoon. But, by 8p.m. we were heading into town for my night out. It went really well; we had a lovely meal and sat and chatted for hours. Well worth the effort of going all the way back for.

One week to go . . .

Thursday

It's all over. No more being a staff nurse. Was my last shift yesterday, I took my remaining leave at the beginning of the shift so I could see my daughter off on her three-day residential school trip. By the time I got in to work at about 10.30a.m. the elective Caesarean section had been done, and I recovered a lady who'd had an instrumental delivery in theatre. We didn't have any emergencies, so I just pottered about stocking up and then spent a relaxing few hours chatting and saying my goodbyes.

It hasn't sunk in yet that I won't be going back there next week . . . am sure it will hit me soon. I know I keep saying it, but I truly love that job, and am really gutted to have left. Although, on the bright side (for me anyway) two more nurses have handed in their notice, so there should be plenty of bank work there soon! I scrubbed for my last section on Monday (not knowing at the time it would be my last) and then on Tuesday I hovered about in theatre whilst a complicated section was performed. The lady had a large cyst growing in one of her ovaries, and after the baby was delivered the surgeons worked to remove the cyst. It was the type of cyst that grows bone, teeth and hair, and when it came out it was enormous. If you can imagine a tub bigger than a large paint pot, but smaller than a bucket . . . the cyst filled it up! It was practically the same size as the baby. I was quite shocked. We put the cyst in the tub to be sent away for testing.

I got my contract from my new Trust at the beginning of the week, and because of the planned postal strike tomorrow I took it to the hospital this morning and hand-delivered it. I am so glad I did, because I was able to get my new ID badge and parking permit at the same time. I now have in my hands my new ID badge, which officially confirms to the world that I am a student midwife. Yippee! I want to wear it everywhere I go so that everybody will know. But that really would be sad!

I had been planning a big BBQ party this Saturday to celebrate becoming a student midwife, and my thirty-first birthday, but the weather has been rubbish so have had to cancel. Instead, I am looking forward to spending the next few days with my family before it all begins!

Friday

Just when I thought I could relax, more drama! After popping all my paperwork into the hospital yesterday, the only thing I had left to do was sort out my uniform. My welcome pack from the hospital had the details, so I rang the sewing room to give them all my measurements as requested. The woman who answered was unsure which uniform I should have, and vaguely confirmed that she thought it was the same as a student nurse . . . great, grey and white stripes for another eighteen months . . . yuk! I was not convinced, so I told her I would ring the uni and then call her back. After speaking to two people who didn't know, I was put through to the lady who interviewed me, who didn't know either. Although she thought it was the same as a staff nurse's uniform, blue and white stripes, better! She was very nice about it all though and suggested I call the midwives directly at the hospital to find out. I rang the midwife who had helped me with my contract, but she wasn't there. Typical!

Well, no rush, don't need a uniform for three weeks yet so I decided to do my housework. Music on full volume, dancing around with the Hoover and the phone rings. Don't know how I heard it, but I did. So I picked it up and could only just hear a lady saying she was a midwifery lecturer from uni . . . ooops . . . not a good first impression with music blaring out full volume! Made my apologies and explained I was doing the housework and turned the music off. She was ringing to find out if I had received a letter confirming the start instructions for Monday. I told her I had; she said a member of my group had phoned advising that she hadn't got it and she was just ringing the rest of us to check we all knew what was happening. While she was on the phone, I asked her about the uniform situation. 'Oh, that's easy,' she said, 'the midwives you will be working with wear scrubs in the hospital and their own clothes in the community.' That's what I had been told originally, months ago . . . good news though, all those clothes I bought and have saved in my wardrobe will now be useful! Mini-drama over. Hopefully there will be no more!

Sunday

Oh my God . . . after all this time it's going to happen tomorrow . . . I have that funny feeling in my stomach, either butterflies, constipation or I don't know what! Am all ready. Bag packed. Clothes ironed (jeans and t-shirt, casual for uni!). Childminder booked. Off for a long soak in the bath . . . and then probably not much sleep!

My Journey as a Student Midwife

Week One

Monday

Have just got home and am knackered. What a day! Didn't sleep much last night; kept waking up. Good job too, because I had set my alarm for 6.45p.m. instead of 6.45a.m. Kids were fantastic this morning and got up and got dressed when I asked them to. They sang me 'Happy Birthday' as I made their packed lunches . . . sweet! Dropped them off at the childminder's at 7.45am and started my drive down the motorway to uni. Realised after five minutes that I was about to run out of petrol, so had to stop to fill up. Traffic was horrendous, took me an hour whereas normally it takes half that, but was rush hour. Never mind, I got there with fifteen minutes to spare.

Had decided to stop smoking today, but nerves got the better of me and I'd had four by the time I walked into uni . . . whoops! Anyway, was told which room to go to and when I got there, one lady was sitting waiting, so I sat down and started chatting to her. A few minutes later we were all there, five of us! Apparently the uni had managed to secure funding for seven places but one person had dropped out, and another hadn't shown up, so it's going to be five of us on this little journey together. Two of the others qualified as nurses six months after me, one about a year before, and the other has been qualified about ten years, so it's a bit of a mixture. We had to do the usual introductions, you know, say a bit about yourself kind-of-thing. The midwifery lecturer showed us some photos of herself through her

27

career and with students she had taught before us, and we chatted and generally got to know each other.

They handed out all our paperwork next. Two huge folders filled with all the assessment paperwork and assignment details, a timetable for the next three weeks, and our ID badges for uni. There was so much paper, the whole process took a couple of hours! Am going to have a good look through it all in a minute; was quite overwhelming.

In the afternoon we had our first lecture, ideologies of maternity/ midwifery care, and we were finished. First day over, so quickly. My back aches from sitting all day. Normally I'm on my feet for twelve and a half hours, although I am sure I won't be complaining after I've been back on placement for a few days! Have had a nice long soak in the bath, and phoned all my family to tell them how I got on and say thank you for all my birthday pressies. One of the girls on my course drives past my house on her way to uni, so we're going to try sharing lifts. She is coming to pick me up tomorrow morning. Will help a lot if we can do this; will halve the money we pay for petrol which will be handy. Am sure I will remember loads more to add, but am truly so tired I can barely type.

Wednesday

I thought they would be gentle with us as newbie student midwives. Boy, was I wrong! Yesterday we had a morning of anatomy, where we were given various diagrams of the vagina and uterus to label. Sounds simple but there are bits down there I never knew I had! Took us all morning to do this, because we also had a workbook to go through where we had to describe the locality and function of various anatomical bits too. We did have a giggle though; none of us knew what a little caterpillar-type looking thing was on one diagram. When our tutor told us it was a clitoris we all fell about laughing. Surely it's men that don't know what that is, not women! The afternoon was easier to digest. We had a lecture about preconception advice; the lecturer was a bit wet. She had us all in stitches unintentionally. We all got the giggles, and that made things worse; we were crying in the end. Guess it's one of those times when you have to be there! She went on and on about how we are what we eat (as one of the girls was chomping through a chocolate bar), how dangerous mobile phones are (we each had ours on silent on the desk in front of us), and how microwaves completely ruin your food. We have decided that next time we have her, we're going to take in a big chocolate cake and microwave popcorn to share, and all sit there talking on our mobile phones when she walks in. Childish, I know!

Today started with a tour of the maternity unit where three of the girls will be based. It looked very dark and dated compared to where I have just been working. Am glad I will not be there. After coffee we had a lecture about communication in midwifery, and then it was on to physiology during pregnancy. This was tough, and again I have come home thinking it will be impossible to learn all this. The lecturer kept reminding us that we had to learn it all for our exam in six months. Only three days in and already the dreaded 'e' word had been mentioned! Four o'clock came, and thankfully it was time to make our ways home, with heads full of hormones and body systems and general feelings of inadequacy at our lack of knowledge. Am going to try and re-read my notes from the lecture and complete the workbook on hormones and their effect on the pregnant woman before going to bed.

Thursday

Went to bed last night with my head swimming with hormones and their effect on the pregnant woman. Was really hard and couldn't finish it all; think I need to spend some more time on it.

Uni was more manageable today. No anatomy and physiology (A&P) . . . hooray! We were given a health promotion task, which involves choosing an area of health promotion related to pregnancy and putting together a presentation to deliver back to the group. I am doing food safety, but am not worrying about it just yet; the presentation is in two weeks and there is other stuff to get through first. Big excitement today; halfway through being told about this presentation the fire alarms went off and we all trooped outside into the car park. After five minutes a fire engine turned up full of firemen (stating the obvious) so we spent the best part of half an hour eyeing them all up. Passed the time!

When we got back inside, we were given a worksheet about embryology which we need to have done by next week . . . more A&P . . . great! It's really in-depth so am going to get it over and done with tonight. What did scare us though was the lecturer telling us that this first lot of A&P is a walk in the park compared to what we have to look forward to. At this point I nearly crawled under the table to cry.

Lectures today were manageable; they focused on woman-centred care and women's sexual health. Both were interesting and easy to follow and we left uni half an hour early. Was hoping to get home in time to collect kids from school but the motorway was at a standstill . . . typical! Still managed to enjoy an hour playing with the children and new rabbit, before making dinner, getting the kids in the bath and putting some washing on. Think I will do the embryology worksheet next then have a bath myself.

Saturday

Hooray . . . have survived the first week! Slept in till 9.30 this morning, must have needed it! Although in my defence I was up till 11p.m. last night preparing a PowerPoint presentation about food safety in pregnancy. Wanted to get it out of the way so I could have the weekend off and not feel guilty. I still have to do some work before Monday, because I only managed to get halfway through the embryology worksheet I attempted on Thursday night. Popped into town this morning and spent some of my birthday money. I treated myself to a large bottle of my favourite perfume, and also invested in a student diary – need to be more organised . . . so hopefully this will help! Spent the afternoon filling in all my uni weeks, placement weeks, clinical assessment and assignment due dates, portfolio days, study days, kids' half-terms, hubby's holidays, looks full already! Oooh, and I got my membership details from the Royal College of Midwives . . . exciting! Haven't had a chance to look through it all yet, but I will! There just doesn't seem to be enough hours in the day anymore. Ooops better go; my son wants to make chocolate cornflake cakes and has been waiting (almost) patiently!

Week Two

Tuesday

We all had another fit of the giggles during our fetal skull and maternal pelvis lecture this afternoon. We were given teaching aids to use, so were all sitting there with models of a fetal skull and maternal pelvis on our desks. The lecturer was happily explaining all the various landmarks on the brim of the pelvis to us when I was nudged in the side by one of the girls. She had got her finger stuck in the foramen magnum hole (the opening for the spinal cord) on her fetal skull! After a lot of pulling it came out with a big pop . . . and that was it, we were all in stitches, laughing so much we were all crying.

We also had a lecture on abdominal palpation. Best lecture yet I think. We went through everything we are going to have to do, and then the lecturer brought in a model of a pregnant female (from neck to groin) and we were able to practise palpating the abdomen and listening to the fetal heart. The model was really clever; she could turn the fetus around, so we didn't know which way it would be lying and you could switch on the fetal heartbeat so we could practise trying to listen to it with a pinard (a small trumpet-like device which midwives use). Cool, loved every minute of it!

Wednesday

Feel like a lump of wobbling jelly today. That's the only way I can describe it. We had a whole day on embryology and to say it was difficult doesn't come close. Just want to curl up in a corner somewhere and cry . . . don't think I will ever get my head round all the different names for the stages of cell division and cell parts. The lecturer must have seen we all felt like this because she finished an hour early. Definitely have brain overload and am not even going to attempt to look at my notes tonight.

Didn't help that kids hadn't wanted to get up and ready this morning. Have been taking them to the childminder's every day between 7.45 a.m. and 8a.m. since I started last week, and it's starting to take its toll. They were tired and irritable, and I got frustrated and shouted, which then made me feel guilty on my drive to uni. Hopefully I will have more self-study time after these first few weeks and then I will be able to take and collect them from school. Managed this during my nursing training, and any study I didn't get done I would finish off in the evenings. We'll see . . .

On a more positive note, we were told that these first three weeks are very intense because we are being given all the information we need to then build on for the next eighteen months. So can only expect it to be like this now, at least I know that things will calm down slightly after this, although by then we will have assignments to write.

Thursday

Got home from uni and was sitting eating tea with hubby and kids when my contact from the hospital rang. She told me that my community placement is going to be in the town next to where I live and who my mentor is going to be. She also confirmed the dates for my first shifts on the delivery suite and the postnatal ward. I am so excited! Hopefully, I will be able to observe a birth on each of my shifts to meet the requirements of my portfolio and then, when I go back to delivery suite for my longer placement, I can get hands-on from the beginning. Not long to wait . . .

Friday

Have had a much deserved day off today . . . managed to get my presentation finished last night so have done nothing midwifery-related at all today, and boy, does it feel good! Never thought I'd be saying that this early on. So, I treated myself, after taking my little boy to the dentist and then dropping him off at school, I went into town to the cinema and watched the new Harry Potter film. Was two hours of pure escapism and I enjoyed having that time to myself. Hubby is working late tonight so instead of cooking tea, we popped to the local chippy and had chips and battered sausage, yummy! Am looking forward to a relaxing weekend, before I'm back at uni on Monday.

Week Three

Monday

Had a lovely weekend, apart from getting drenched in a thunderstorm with my daughter when walking the dog . . . never mind, she thought it was a huge adventure! Back at uni today and we did the first stage of labour, which was really interesting, think we all enjoyed it. Kids had sports day at school, but I wasn't able to get back in time to cheer them on. Was gutted, never missed one before . . .

Tuesday

Was the dreaded presentation day today! All went quite well really, even with my nerves I managed to get through it OK. Although I didn't attempt to pronounce some of the longer very complicated words . . . Ha ha ha . . .

Also managed to get my usernames and password sorted out for home access to the universities' digital library. Will be much-needed in a couple of weeks when I have to start the assignments that all seem to be due in on the same day in a couple of months' time! Can feel the pressure starting to pile on, what with knowing I have to complete four assignments, a clinical portfolio, choose women for my caseload, get to grips with working in the community, hospital orientation, theory days at uni and prepare for the exam. Don't think I will have much time for anything at all for the next six months. I know they said it was a full-on course but this is REALLY full-on!

Thursday

Fabulous day. We covered second and third stages of labour today. Was really good fun. We had to pretend to be the fetus going through the pelvic cavity by lying on the floor and emerging in the correct way by twisting and turning our heads, necks and bodies from under a table. Made us laugh so much I got cramp, quickly followed by a carpet burn on my arm when my descent was too fast.

We were all given pagers today. We have to staple our pager numbers to the handheld notes of the women we caseload, and choose to follow through their pregnancies so when they go into labour we are able to be contacted and can meet them at hospital or their home to deliver their babies. Spent a good hour trying to work out how to use mine, but managed it in the end.

Not in uni tomorrow, we have a study day for next week's presentation. Mine is on the drugs which women can safely take whilst breastfeeding. Has worked out really well because tomorrow is also the children's last day at school before the summer holidays, so I will be able to take them and pick them up. Then I have the weekend off, and will start with my community midwife on Monday. She phoned me last night, and although she wasn't horrible, she sounded rather stressed so am a bit apprehensive about meeting her. Am sure it will be fine, but could have done without that added worry.

Week Four

Monday

Have just got home from my first day out in the community as a student midwife . . . and it was amazing! I love it. Got to the GP practice at 8.45a.m. and none of the midwives were there. After about ten minutes two of them arrived, and both are lovely (don't know what I was so worried about).

They had their monthly meeting with the health visitor first, which involved discussing the women on the caseload who needed extra support. After a quick cup of tea we were off to do our first visit. It was a booking visit and we pulled up outside a rather posh-looking house. I couldn't wait to get in and get started! The husband answered the door and let us in, and as soon as I stepped through the door I recognised the wife and said hello (we had worked previously together when I was a student nurse). This caused a rather heated discussion between the husband and my mentor. He was angry that they hadn't been told a student was coming, and that I was someone who knew his wife because they hadn't told anyone that she was expecting. My mentor tried to defuse the situation and advised him that I was unable to tell anyone due to confidentiality, but that didn't seem to help. I felt awful; not a good start unfortunately. Things calmed down and eventually I was invited to stay, although the atmosphere remained incredibly tense. As I had not seen a booking being completed before

I sat and listened to everything my mentor was saying. It was a lot of information, not sure I'll be able to remember all this! Back out in the car I apologised to my mentor, who was lovely and said it wasn't my fault, but it didn't make me feel any better.

We then had three postnatal home visits to do, and I was thrown straight in at the deep end and did them all myself. It basically involves doing a head to toe check on Mum and her baby, and talking through any concerns the new parents might have, answering any questions and offering lots of advice. After watching a heel prick test (the neonatal screening blood test) I did the second one myself, and managed it (just!). By this time it was getting on for 1p.m. and we met another midwife for lunch at a garden centre.

As soon as I was introduced, she said she recognised me from when I had done my elective placement at the hospital as a student nurse. I said I was sorry but I couldn't place her. It slowly dawned on me who she was . . . it was once again the midwife who had been called in to help deliver my placenta when my son was born! That was the third time our paths had crossed. She was very welcoming and will definitely be supportive as I progress through the course.

After lunch, we had another booking appointment and one final postnatal check and then we were back to the GP practice. I had a chance to show my mentor my portfolio and she signed the bits I needed her to. I didn't complete any of my portfolio today, although I could have done. Thought I'd spend a couple of days just settling in, although with an antenatal clinic tomorrow I think I will make an effort to get started.

I really need to get my caseload women sorted out as soon as possible. I have to caseload five women, which means I have to complete their booking at the beginning of the pregnancy, see them antenatally a minimum of five times, care for them in labour and deliver their baby, and visit them postnatally a couple of times. The advice from uni is that we caseload a lot more than five women, just in case any of them miscarry or deliver without us being there. So the plan is to caseload around fifteen. The logistics of seeing these women at the correct times is going to be complicated, but I'll worry about that when I need to!

Managed to complete my second presentation on breastfeeding and medication over the weekend, so am looking forward to an evening of reading the last Harry Potter book (am already halfway through, it's fab!). Will also spend some time on the phone ringing the others in my group to hear all about their first days.

Wednesday

Had antenatal clinics all day today. The morning was really good. My main mentor is fabulous, pushing me to get in there and take over from her. So after watching her do one lady, I did the rest – with her help. Was practising my abdominal palpations, using the sonic aid to locate the fetal heartbeat and I did all the writing in the ladies' hand-held notes. We finished about 1.45p.m. My main mentor had the afternoon off because she is on-call tonight. We agreed that she would only ring me if there were something interesting happening, because if I were to go on-call with her and nothing happened, then I would be down on my required hours. So she left and I worked with my second mentor for the afternoon; she too was doing an antenatal clinic and I thought it would be more opportunity to get some experience . . . not the case . . . not the case at all. She works very differently and had me sitting the other side of the room watching her all afternoon. She occasionally asked the ladies if I could have a feel of their tummies, and I did the odd urine dipstick but apart from that, nothing.

The bad thing is my mentor is going off on holiday for two weeks and therefore I will be working with my second mentor for the whole time. Am not looking forward to it at all. Only saving grace is that next week I have three days' orientation at the hospital, so that leaves just two days with her. Trying not to be negative, but just can't help feeling like I will be losing out on lots of learning experiences . . . will just have to try and make the most of it. It's not that she's a nasty person – quite the opposite, she's lovely – it's just the way she works with a student that's a bit jarring.

Thursday

Did my first booking today, all by myself. Well, nearly . . . mentor stepped in a few times, just to jog my memory when I stumbled a bit! But all in all it went very well. The advice she gave me afterwards was not to talk too much in depth about anti-d immunoglobulin (if a woman has rhesus negative blood type then this is an injection offered to them at 28 weeks gestation), and to ensure I look to see if the woman is working, as she may need advice on what time off she is due for her antenatal appointments and maternity leave etc. Feel proud that I managed it though!

We also did a parentcraft class this evening. Tonight's class was at the hospital and it was basically showing a group of expectant mums and their partners round the delivery suite and postnatal ward. I wasn't much use, having not worked there for over a year (and then only for a month) so I just stayed in the background and observed. Felt slightly uncomfortable when I had to introduce myself to thirty complete strangers, always turn a deep tomato-red colour. Hope I can get used to speaking in front of so many people!

Friday

Back at uni today. Was lovely to see the others and hear about how they have been getting on. We all had stories to tell, and spent the morning chatting and learning about reflection (the basis of an essay we have to do). The rest of the day was spent talking this over and getting some advice from our lecturer about the layout of the essay and what is expected for a degree-level assignment (scary!).

Week Five

Monday

Have had a lovely weekend, with visits from my dad, and then my brother and nephew too. Got all the boring housie jobs done as well; washing, cleaning, ironing etc. Didn't do anything midwifery, although I feel justified by my choice as I was up till 1a.m. Friday night trawling the Internet for statistics I need for my first assignment which I have now started . . . It's in the research and planning stages anyway.

Have my first shift on delivery suite today, am working a late shift, which is 1.30p.m. to 9.30p.m. and I am starting to feel a bit nervous. Hope I get to observe a birth! Just have those horrible first-day worries. Where do I go? Where are the scrubs? Where is the changing room? Is there a fridge for my pack-up? What will people be like? I know it's a little easier for me, as I spent a month there last year, but I still feel very anxious.

Tuesday

Last two days have been fabulous! Yesterday was really exciting! All the midwives were really welcoming and made me feel comfortable and at ease when I arrived for my first shift as a student midwife on delivery suite. The midwife I worked with was the same midwife I had spent a week with as a student nurse, so it was nice to see her and catch up. She had done the same as me, worked as a nurse for ten months and then started her midwifery training, and has now been working as a midwife for a couple of years. We were given the care of a lady having her third baby (gravida three para two in midwifery-speak – see, am getting the hang of this lark already!!). Her first baby had been by emergency section for breech presentation and her second baby had been a forceps delivery. When we entered the room, she was immaculately made-up and looked very comfortable. She was labouring

39

without any pain relief and made it all look so easy. She was due an examination to check her dilation – my mentor did this and then announced with a huge grin that she was fully dilated and ready to start pushing! And off she went, pushing with such determination that it was incredible to watch. Then came her Jekyll and Hyde moment where she switched repeatedly from being calm and controlled to being absolutely manic. It was at this point my mentor offered her some Entonox (gas and air) to help her through (we had offered it previously but she had refused). She used the Entonox at the start of each contraction and then pushed. Gradually I could see an odd wrinkled blue lump emerging from her. The lump got larger and larger. I looked at my mentor in pure horror trying to work out exactly what I was looking at, worried that I was about to witness the birth of Frankenstein Junior, but she looked as calm and serene as ever. I was left guessing that this was in fact normal so I tried to mask the look of utter confusion with an encouraging smile! After forty-five minutes of pushing, the large blue wrinkled lump suddenly became longer, and then with a pop the baby's face was there, looking down at the bed and then turning to look directly at me. Two large eyes were gazing at me, and then blinked very slowly! The large blue lumpy thing that had confused me so much was the back of the baby's head . . . seemed so obvious in retrospect. With the next push a gorgeous baby boy was born to my pure delight, and of course that of his mum and dad. He gurgled, then cried for a matter of seconds and then just stared at us all with his huge eyes. Was an amazing and very special moment.

Our second lady of the shift was a first time mum who had been labouring at home but was now finding it too much. My mentor said we would assess her, but not to expect another birth because first time mums always labour longer – famous last words! She had a history of her waters breaking and having contractions every couple of minutes. We popped her onto the CTG machine because it had been twenty-four hours since her waters broke, and this let us monitor the baby's heart rate and her contractions simultaneously. Her contractions were coming four in every ten minutes and the baby was coping very well. We helped her relax and showed her how to use the Entonox. After what felt like five minutes but was probably more like an hour, she started to involuntarily push at the peak of her contractions. My mentor winked at me and nodded towards the door, I followed her out of the room and she explained that our lady was probably in the transitional phase and may well be fully dilated already. We went back into the room and during her next contraction, we peeked under the sheets and to my complete surprise I could see the now-familiar sight of a lumpy blue wrinkled baby's head! We told her this and she was off! Pushing like a real trooper. There had been a little meconium (a baby's first bowel movement) in her waters so another midwife had been called into the room for the birth. It had only been slight and my mentor said it was nothing to worry about. It took her a good hour to push the baby out. Finally the baby's head was born and restituted very quickly (moved to re-align with baby's shoulders). Baby was OP (occipito posterior, where the baby's spine is against the mother's spine, so the head is facing upwards), so was looking up at us; the shoulders were delivered and the rest followed, along with a lot of very black sticky meconium. Baby was put onto Mum's chest for a cuddle and I helped to rub all the meconium from his little body, but he didn't cry and was turning a horrible colour (very quickly). The second midwife scooped him up, popped him onto the Resuscitaire and started frantically rubbing him. We were all willing him to breathe. Mum was crying, Dad was pale and in a stunned silence, and we were all very worried. The emergency button had been pulled and the senior midwife was in the room before we knew it. Paeds (paediatricians) had also been called. Baby was suctioned and given oxygen, then finally spluttered out a cry. All was OK. In a more relaxed atmosphere the placenta was delivered, and then the paed arrived, just a little late!

My mentor and I had stayed beyond our shift to deliver this little boy (because it was busy, there was a shortage of midwives on the night shift and more importantly because we had bonded with Mum and Dad and wanted to be there for them), but the midwife taking over was happy to clear up and take over so we left. We did pop in and see them on the postnatal ward today and they were preparing to go home with their gorgeous little boy!

Today didn't bring me any more births but I did enjoy my shift. We cared for a first time mum who had an epidural set up and had a drug called Syntocinon (Synto) running through a drip to help regulate and strengthen her contractions. She was lovely, so was her husband, and we popped in and out of the room most of the shift checking her CTG. She was still going strong when I left at 3.30p.m. so fingers crossed she will have her little baby by now! We also cared for another first time mum who had come in because her waters had broken and her contractions were becoming more regular. I took the lead with this one, did the assessment and popped her on the CTG just to monitor how things were going. She was fine, although her contractions were still really irregular, so we advised her to go home and establish into labour, and if things hadn't kicked off overnight then to come back to delivery suite in the morning so baby could be checked.

In the middle of all this, I also helped (very briefly) care for a woman post C-section. Her midwife was baby-catching for another section and she needed someone to check her obs (observations) regularly. I found this quite hard, because the way this Trust do things is slightly different from what I'm used to, but I just did as I was told and got on with it! The level of care was the same (top-notch, obviously) and I'm sure I will come across that a lot; will just take a while to get used to how things are done here. Am knackered now, after working a late and then an early and I now have two days in the community with the second mentor to deal with, and I'm dreading it. If things don't improve I will speak to my personal tutor at uni for advice. I haven't touched my assignment since Friday night, so I now have that horrible niggling feeling that I should be getting on with it. Will try and get some info from second mentor tomorrow; she is the teenage pregnancy queen and this is what I have decided to base my essay on, so maybe I will earn some brownie points that way. Worth a try!

Friday

Had a roller-coaster few days. Worked with second mentor Wednesday and Thursday. Wednesday started off very badly, mentor spent most of the morning huffing and puffing about having a student and how awful it was. Felt like getting up and walking out but why should I give up all that I have achieved just because of her attitude? Persevered anyway, and at lunchtime we started getting on – couldn't quite believe it! Then it was happy times. She was involving me more in her post-natal visits, and then let me do a couple of the antenatal clinic appointments myself. On Thursday we did a parentcraft class together (three-hour session) and we were a team, it was really good. Amazingly she even apologised for her behaviour, and now seems to have really taken me under her wing. Because my main mentor is on holiday still next week and I am scheduled to work in the community all next week, she has arranged other things for me to do when she is not on duty. She is doing a shift on delivery suite next Friday and has said she wants me to go with her so I can hopefully get my first hands-on delivery! It's fantastic; feel so much better now.

Today I did my orientation shift on the postnatal ward, and again I had a really good day. I observed a postnatal mum and baby check, and then I did three myself, and generally tried to help out where I could. One of the midwives was called to delivery because they were full and didn't have enough midwives, so that left the ward one midwife down, but we coped . . . although we didn't get a break. Have filled in more of my portfolio and I have arranged to spend Monday morning on the day assessment unit (DAU) so I will be able to gain some experience caring for antenatal women who have high-risk pregnancies. I know I keep saying it, but am not doing any midwifery stuff this weekend. Have worked full-time all week and spent two (long) evenings working on my essay, so am just going to chill.

Week Six

Tuesday

Had fab day in community, antenatal clinic in the morning and post-natal visits in the afternoon, only to come home to a letter from my childminder. She has given me four weeks' notice of not having my kids anymore . . . great. She says my little boy is too difficult to handle, and she is getting complaints from the other parents about his behaviour. I know he can be a handful, and is full of energy and very stubborn, but what she won't accept is that he comes home crying most days because the other kids she looks after and her 'angel' of a daughter have been bullying him. Should have moved him somewhere else ages ago, but it was easy to keep him there because she was flexible. This now seems like such a lame reason to continue using her, and makes me feel like such a bad mother, but it's over now and anyway it's kind of a relief. I have got the phone number for the before and after school club which I am going to try, and hopefully my sister-in-law will be able to have them through the holidays. Just feel guilty now that I am out full-time doing my training when perhaps I should be at home with them. But this conversion course is the last one that is being run, and if I don't do it now, I may never have the chance again. It's what I have wanted for so long. I took my little lad for a walk with the dog when I got home from work and we had a long chat (he's eight, so understands things to a certain extent) and he says he is happy that he doesn't have to go back to the childminder. Just praying that my sister-in-law will agree to the school holidays! It's a horrid feeling, being torn between kids and midwifery and the guilt and feelings of being selfish are yukky . . . hope we can get through this OK.

Wednesday

Feeling better today. Spent the whole day doing antenatal clinics, oh the joy! Was good fun, practised palpating abdomens and using sonic aids, also got to grips with using the computer to record consultations. On the downside, I ended up looking at haemorrhoids and taking a vaginal swab because of smelly green discharge (nice!). Have got a booking to do tomorrow and going to a case conference about a pregnant lady who is an alcoholic which will be very sad, but also it should be interesting from a learning perspective. Will let you know.

Hubby and kids go on holiday tomorrow. Feeling down about that because I haven't really been separated from the kids like that before. We always go on holiday as a family (and spend the whole time arguing), but it's still horrible that I can't go. Will keep in touch by phone and will be joining them for the weekend, but it's still not the same.

Friday

Feeling lonely! Not used to having the house to myself. Have been in touch with kids and they are having a lovely time. I will be joining them tomorrow for the weekend, so can't wait for that!

Did an early today on delivery with my second community mentor. She didn't have a clue . . . she was like a fish out of water, was rather amusing to watch actually! In the community she knows her stuff, but on delivery . . . well, can only describe it as an excruciating shift! We cared for a first time mum who was in spontaneous labour. She got to fully dilated within a couple of hours and was coping on Entonox. She started her second stage at 10.30a.m. and my mentor said to expect baby by 11a.m. All was going brilliantly, except she couldn't seem to shift the baby. To cut a long story short, my first hands-on delivery ended up being an episiotomy/forceps delivery done by the doctor. I was gutted for the woman, as she had worked so hard, and selfishly I was gutted for myself because I had worked so hard too. But her little boy was born, nice and healthy, and we were all smiles that he had arrived. Had started at 7.30a.m. and finished at 3.30p.m. without a break and am feeling knackered to say the least!

My father-in-law has taken pity on me being here on my own and has invited me round for dinner (prawn curry, my favourite!) and then I will do another couple of hours on my essay which is half done now, thanks to all the evenings I have been putting in collecting statistics and research.

Only two days left with second mentor, and then my own mentor is back from her hols, so can't wait to get going with her again.

Week Seven

Wednesday

Had a fabulous weekend camping with kids! Needed it, to relax and de-stress. Kids are sorted too, daughter is off to my mum's next week and son is booked into a kids' activity summer camp. Just got to sort out the week after now. Both are booked into before and after school club, so am glad to have got all that arranged.

The week in the community so far has been amazing. I can feel my confidence growing day by day. My second mentor practically let me run the antenatal clinic, and that really made me feel useful. She said she had no worries about me, as I was managing well, and giving good advice! Fab! My main mentor returned from her holiday today, but I only spent a couple of hours with her in the morning and then carried on with second mentor for the afternoon. Am looking forward to being back at uni tomorrow and catching up with the other girls.

Week Eight

Monday

Have learnt so much in last few days. I am back with my main mentor and I am so glad. She gets me to do the visits etc. and will just chip in if I miss anything or ask for her advice. It's great! She was on-call over the weekend, and we went out to a lady who had a history of her first delivery being very fast. She reported having contractions and feeling baby's head was between her legs! So we went flying round there but it was all a false alarm. She wasn't in labour, we did a thorough antenatal check and asked if she would consent to a vaginal examination (VE), which she did and my mentor found she had a non-labouring cervix. She had also consented to me repeating the examination. It was my first VE and I was so frightened of doing it. I think I felt the cervix, although, being completely honest I'm not entirely sure what the hell I was feeling. At least I got the first one over with . . . the others won't seem so bad now I hope!!

Sunday was spent visiting, and again I led all the visits, and mentor just added bits as and when necessary. We did my formative assessment, which I passed! Hooray, first assessment out the way! Then I took my daughter to my mum's where she is staying for the week and spent some time with my little boy, which was nice, we read books and had a cuddle, just some mummy and son time together.

Back at work today with second mentor, who was in a particularly foul mood. She didn't let me do anything, it's sooo frustrating. Total waste of time actually. What is her problem? We finished at 2.30p.m. and I am home already, so am going to make the best use of the time and try and get some more of my assignment done. It seems to be going very slowly . . .

Friday

Have nearly finished my assignment . . . at last!! Am over the word count so need to go back and chop bits out, but at least the majority of it has been done. Plan to email it to my tutor next week. She can't read it all; apparently they are permitted to read 10% of it, but just want her to have a quick look and tell me if I have missed out anything major.

Community has been good. Tuesday I was on delivery suite, did a couple of VEs, even managed to feel cervical dilatation and the baby's head, but couldn't feel sutures so was unsure of the position of the baby, but I have been promised that it will come with time. Neither of the ladies I cared for had vaginal deliveries though. Am set to be the high-risk queen I think! The first lady seemed to be having progressively stronger contractions but when we VE'd her after four hours to assess her progress in labour there was no change, so she ended up on a Syntocinon drip with an epidural, and had not delivered when I left (an hour after my shift had finished). The other lady I was caring for had an unreassuring CTG and the consultant was called. She had an emergency C-section (I've seen enough of them already!).

Have had plenty of opportunities to practise antenatal and postnatal care in the community. My main mentor is on-call tonight and just as we were finishing at 5p.m. we heard that a planned home birth lady had called to say she was in labour. Her local midwife was on the way and phoned us shortly afterwards to say that she was 2cm dilated and progressing well, so am now sitting at home waiting for the call to go out and (fingers crossed) deliver her baby! Have been trying to keep busy and not just watch the phone. Have been out and trimmed all the bushes in the front garden, which were so overgrown you couldn't see the house number on the wall. So annoying when people don't have a house number you can see! Speaking from experience here from the frustrating times I have had as a student midwife on community placement, trying to find houses with no numbers on them!

Rang daughter who is at Mum's. She sounded very homesick and

I can't wait to see her tomorrow. My little boy has had an amazing time at the activity club over the last week, and is desperate to go back again next year (such a relief). Also had a chat with fellow student midwife on the phone last night. She had taken blood for the first time in years and we both laughed when she said she had been so nervous she was shaking. Luckily the woman having her blood taken had been looking the other way so hadn't seen the shaking needle heading towards her. Anyway, will let you know how tonight goes!

Week ten

Sunday

Home birth the other week unfortunately didn't result in my first catch. The woman was just about coping, and she wanted to know how she was progressing, so we did a VE. In the four hours since her last VE, her cervix hadn't dilated any further at all. This was a really big shock to us all, as she seemed to have been having strong regular contractions. Anyhow, she made the decision to go into hospital for stronger pain relief so I was home by 11.30p.m. Worked with my mentor the next day and we popped into the hospital to see her; she had ended up with a forceps delivery at around breakfast time.

Last week was a complete and utter waste of time . . . rubbish in fact. Trust induction. Disaster from start to finish. The programme I had was all wrong; they kept changing the times at the last minute. I ended the week sixteen hours down on what I should have done, due to stupid two- or three-hour sessions slap-bang in the middle of the day, so I was unable to work before or after as my mentor could have been anywhere in the surrounding area. Friday I was only there for forty-five minutes. Stupid. Feel like I have wasted a whole week.

Have received an email from my personal tutor saying my essay is very well written. Hooray!!! She gave me some useful comments, and I am still working on it. Have also started my reflection essay, and hope to have that done this week, in-between having my hair done on Wednesday and hopefully observing a post-mortem on Friday (to help with my anatomy and physiology exam). But back to uni tomorrow for the research module . . . yikes! I hate research, and got my lowest grade (B) for my research essay as a student nurse. Not looking forward to it much, but can't wait to see the others and have a good old natter. The three-year direct entry student midwives start tomorrow too, and a couple of them used to be HCAs where I used to work, so will be keeping an eye out for them to give them some moral support on their first day.

Week Eleven

Wednesday

Doing the research module this week, and to say it's gone straight in one ear and out the other is an understatement. It's hard, boring and I just feel like banging my head against a brick wall. We had three hours of lectures about quantitative research critiquing today and it was all $x = p + n$ . . . blah blah blah! Didn't get it, don't think I ever will. Tried to look intelligent and nod in all the right places but don't think I fooled anyone! Only saving grace is that we can choose to critique a qualitative study for our research essay, still hard, but think it might be the easier option, so no guessing what I will be doing then.

Private study day today and I have used my time very constructively. Spent three hours at my neighbour's having my hair coloured and cut. Then had to pop to town to change my little boy's school shoes because after only five days of wearing them, they had fallen apart . . . must be a new record I think! Anyway, am going to try and finish my reflective assignment tonight, and have planned to spend the next private study day (Friday) rather more productively in the library getting references to add in here and there.

Week Thirteen

Thursday

Don't know where to start really. Have been through it a bit the last couple of weeks. Reached the point where I was actually going to quit. Even phoned my old work to beg my manager for my job back but she wasn't there at the time.

Research week was awful. Just found it hard to grasp the concepts, and understand all the terminology being used. Can't find a qualitative research study to critique, but am trying not to dwell on that. Whilst trying to cope with that, my son decided to really misbehave himself. Got to crisis point and I rang the school nurse asking for help to try and manage his difficult behaviour. She promised to speak to the school and the school doctor and get back to me, but she hasn't yet. Have started a reward chart, but got home from uni today to find he has been given a yellow card for throwing conkers at school, and he was being told off for silly behaviour at after school club when I picked him up. So . . . have again been struggling with the guilt of not being at home to look after him, and also with my own feelings of wanting to be a midwife so much, that now I have finally made it on to the course, I just can't give it all up. Rubbish.

On top of all that I have written two assignments and still have one more to do, plus our exam is coming up in a few months' time, and I have a research essay to write, and a dissertation proposal to put together. Really feeling the pressure . . . maybe it wasn't a good idea to try and do a midwifery degree in eighteen months. Everything just seems to have snowballed and suddenly become too much. Sounds lame when I read it back, but feeling guilty, crying all the time and still having to cope with uni, kids, miserable husband and house is bloody hard work. Sometimes I feel like walking . . .

Had quite a heavy day with anatomy and physiology (A&P) at uni today. One of the girls walked out of the lecture in tears, she just couldn't cope with the pressure of the complicated A&P, essays, and the exam . . . I know exactly how she feels! Hoping things will calm down over the next ten days. Tomorrow is a study day, and then I have next week as annual leave. Although I have to go through the two essays already written to check all the references, and write the third from scratch. Have a blood test at the new Trust to prove that I am Hep B, Hep C and HIV negative . . . and then the good bits are an Ann Summers party to go and get legless at, meeting with the girls I did my nursing training with, and meeting up with one of the girls I used to work in theatres with. Will need another week off to get over my week off at this rate.

Week Fifteen

Thursday

Been a while since I made an entry in my journal . . . oops, just don't have enough time these days! Had a lovely week's holiday; well, sort of – nothing is ever simple!! Was planning on finishing off all my assignments, did finish two, and then the next morning I woke up to find that my phone line was faulty and I had no Internet access. Rang the phone company on my mobile and waited in a queue for thirty minutes whilst a positively annoying woman kept telling me to report my fault online because it was quicker – typical. Well, if I had Internet access I would bloody report my fault online, however the reason I was ringing was to report my phone line and therefore Internet faulty . . . Aaarrrggghhh. When I finally spoke to a human being I was told that it would be at least a week before it was fixed, something about rural phone lines . . . blah blah blah . . . frustrating! Ended up popping into uni (forty-mile round trip) to get the stuff off the Internet that I needed.

Then, on Thursday I had to pop to occupational health, they wanted to take blood to confirm my measles immunity. Had blood test and went and sorted off-duty for delivery suite (another story I will fill you in on in a mo), and drove home. On the way home my arm really started to hurt, but being a nurse an aching arm wasn't going to cause me any concern so I just ignored it. Thought I'd have a cuppa when I got back; tea is the answer to everything, even aching arms. Now, I have to admit that I started to feel a little alarmed when I tried and failed to pick the kettle up because my arm was hurting so much, and couldn't believe it when I saw that I had a haematoma the size of a tennis ball where the blood had been taken! I got back in my car, and managed to drive to my doctor's surgery. When I got there I showed the receptionist my arm and she hurried me into see a doctor straight-away. The doctor confirmed it was a haematoma (doh . . .) and advised to put a cold compress on it and wait for it to come out in a bruise. That was it, no words of medical wisdom that I wasn't already aware of myself. Only thing was I couldn't move my bloody arm at all, so couldn't do anything, no housework, but more importantly no assign-ment (crap!). So I spent the last two days of my week's holiday sitting on the sofa feeling sorry for myself, with my arm balanced on cushions, with no phone to even take my mind off the pain by nattering to friends. A week later and I have a bruise like you have never seen, my whole arm from shoulder to wrist is a splendid combination of blues, greens and yellows and it's still uncomfortable sleeping. Moral of the story, don't let occupational health staff take your blood.

Did have some good news though, I have been paid at a lower band than I should have been for the last six months, and I am due to have it all backdated! Hooray!! Only found out when I phoned them to query it . . . bloody NHS for you.

Back to my off-duty for delivery suite. I rang during my week's holiday (before the phone went faulty) and my mentor just happened to answer the phone. She gave me her off-duty for the next three weeks and asked if it was OK for me to shadow her shifts so we could get to know each other properly. Her shifts are awful. My first week there she's on holiday, but was kind enough to arrange for me to work with someone else. The following two weeks she's on nights . . . six nights . . . It's going to kill me! It's not that I don't enjoy nights, it's that my body doesn't handle it very well, and I end up not knowing what day it is and whether I should be eating breakfast at 6p.m. when I am getting up and dinner at 9a.m. when I am going to bed. It's going to be an experience anyway.

So, back to this week. Had Monday off. Tuesday was uni; revising the mechanisms of labour. Two of the girls went straight to placement on delivery suite from uni (nasty off-duty), and I got a text from one later that evening to say she had got her first catch! Yesterday was my first shift back on delivery suite. Was just walking through the doors and my community mentor was there; she said she was hoping to catch me as one of my caseload ladies had delivered her twins at twenty-two weeks (they hadn't survived), and she wanted to be sure I knew. Poor lady.

Delivery suite was empty, only three labouring women there and all very early on (4cm dilated). Not looking good for my first hands-on delivery! Worked with a lovely midwife and we cared for a first time mum who was coping beautifully. Had a good feeling about this one. Mentor did VE four hours after the last one and there had been no further progress. Also fresh red blood loss now. Lady was reviewed by doctor, plan was for Synto infusion to be started and the baby to be monitored on a CTG. To cut a long story short, the baby didn't like the stronger contractions and infusion was on, off, on, off . . . we handed her over to the night staff at 9.30p.m. My mentor said she expected her to end up with a C-section if she continued not to make progress (we had done another VE and dilatation had remained the same all day).

So, I got home last night, knackered, and disappointed that yet again I had not delivered a baby. Had a bowl of cereal and went to bed. Had to get up to get the kids to school this morning and feel absolutely shattered. Have had a quick whizz round, shoving laundry in washing machine and then tumble dryer, filled dishwasher and am about to sit down with a nice cup of tea and watch trashy daytime TV. Am on a late again today followed by an early tomorrow (late shift followed by an early shift, yuk!), so start at 1.30p.m. and hospital is very close by so will leave here about 1p.m. Fingers crossed again that I get my first delivery, although I am not holding my breath.

Friday

I did it! At last! My first hands-on delivery happened last night at 7.15p.m., a beautiful little girl weighing in at 2777g (6lb 2oz), and I had looked after my lady on my own (under the supervision of a senior midwife). She had arrived on delivery suite having strong regular contractions, coping brilliantly. I supported her, and felt confident listening in to the baby's heartbeat every fifteen minutes. At 6.45p.m. the baby's heart rate had a deceleration to 95–100bpm (beats per minute) and I immediately informed my mentor, who came in to the room. Her next contraction saw baby's heart rate drop again, this time to 70bpm . . . and midwife in charge was called, who bleeped for the doctors. By now my lady was pushing with everything she had to get baby out. All of a sudden her little head emerged, followed by her body (obviously!) and I caught little one, and put her on Mum's tummy. Just as the doctors were walking into the room all was good. Mum and baby fine. Was amazing! Checked baby had the correct number of fingers and toes, and that everything was in the right place whilst mentor sutured a little perineal tear. Was perfect! Came home on a real high!

Didn't feel quite so good when I had to get up at 6a.m. to start the early shift today at 7.30a.m. Board was chock-a-block full on delivery (the board is where all details of labouring mums are written). Had handover and was given a multip (had one or more babies already) to look after, who was feeling pushy. Sounded promising, so off I trotted into the room with my mentor and before even having a chance to say 'hello', my mentor had handed me some gloves and was pushing me round the bed getting me into catching position! Within a few minutes I had caught a gorgeous little boy . . . catch number two! His shoulders had been transverse as his body delivered, and Mum had a tear that needed suturing, so while my mentor did that I weighed and checked baby, labelling him up with his little ankle bands and giving him his jab of vitamin K (this is offered to all newborn babies to help with their blood clotting, so it basically helps reduce the risk of them bleeding internally). Then I checked the placenta and membranes, all appeared complete. Baby breastfed like a star, and when he was finished I helped Mum walk across to the shower before we transferred her and her new baby across to the ward.

Got back to delivery (which was still very busy at this point) and was allocated the care of a lady having an elective C-section. Mentor had already completed pre-op checklist, and we popped her on the monitor (CTG) for a bit because Mum's blood pressure was high. Went into theatre with her, scrubbed, received the baby, little boy, gave vitamin K, did baby check, and recovered Mum post-operatively.

All in all has been a fabulous day, although not when I got back home and went to the after school club to get the kids. Bearing in mind I hadn't seen them since taking them to school yesterday morning, I thought they would be really excited to see me, but no . . . Little boy burst into tears at seeing me, and said he wanted to stay and play at club for a bit longer. Talk about feeling disappointed! Least I know he likes club though, much better than when they were with child-minder when they were both desperate to get home. He has a cub sleepover tonight, so just getting ready to take him there now. Looking forward to having a day off tomorrow, then I will be working an early again on Sunday.

Sunday

Stayed up late watching a film last night and did not want to get up when the alarm went off at 6a.m.! Got to delivery suite and only one lady was in labour; my mentor and I were given her to care for. She was a multip who had been induced for essential hypertension (high blood pressure). She had the full whack of Synto running through a drip but was only contracting one in ten (one in every ten minutes). She also had an epidural, so I was able to practise my VEs, which was fab. First VE I felt she was 8cms dilated, and could feel suture line in direct OP position. At the second VE she was exactly the same; consultant came in and it was decided she should have a Caesarean section. So I caught the baby at that. No-one else in labour came in, so had the chance to do all the paperwork for section, and fill in my portfolio with mentor.

Came home, absolutely knackered and little boy wanted to go on a bike ride. Off we went . . . three miles! Legs felt like jelly when we finally got home again. Have just cooked and eaten Sunday dinner, put kids in the bath and then to bed, had a bath myself and I am now off to bed too. It's only 7.30p.m. Sad, or what? Thankfully I have Monday and Tuesday off, although I will carry on working on my essays, which are nearly finished. Back in the community on Wednesday and then I start my run of two weeks' worth of nights.

Week Eighteen

Monday

Am knackered. Have done all six of my nights, finished at 8a.m. this morning and have managed to sleep for four hours. Will be getting an early night though, as doing an early tomorrow.

It's been a wonderful two weeks. Have now caught seven babies! Seven! Had a couple of scary moments. One woman laboured so quickly that the baby was born rather congested and the paeds had to be called; resuscitation was required. Another came in, she was a para two, so had given birth to two babies previously and had a history of quick deliveries. She looked so calm and collected, my mentor (outside of the room) said she didn't think she was in labour. We did a quick CTG (she was only thirty-six weeks gestation) and as I was writing up the CTG at the midwives' station, her buzzer went. We went into the room and she very calmly whispered that the head was coming. We had a look and sure enough, there was the head! Just managed to get my gloves on as the head crowned and a beautiful little girl arrived very gracefully into the world. Had us all surprised!

Also had a drama one night when we took a call from a paramedic who was en route with a labouring twins lady (thirty-seven weeks gestation). A few minutes later, A&E were calling frantically requesting we get down to them quickly. The babies had both been born breech in the back of the ambulance, and delivered by the poor paramedic! I was told to grab the emergency bag, a suitcase on wheels with all our kit in it, and we ran full tilt along the hospital corridors, down the stairs and into A&E. You could see the look of relief on the nurses' faces when we burst through the door. No-one had the common sense to wrap these tiny twins up to keep them warm, so I grabbed one and my mentor grabbed the other and we started bundling them up in towels until they looked like little caterpillar cocoons with faces just visible. Mum was absolutely fine, so she was transferred to delivery suite where she delivered the placenta. Both babies were perfect in every way, just gave us all a heart-stopping moment. (Note to self; start jogging. Being just a little bit fitter might well come in handy as a midwife!)

Last night I cared for a lovely lady who was not progressing very quickly. She was on the CTG machine as she had prolonged rupture of membranes, and had a Synto infusion. She was given pethidine for pain relief at around 8.30 that evening and was coping well, although the baby was not very active. All seemed OK, and we got her an epidural so she could doze for a while, and I popped a urinary catheter in. My mentor went for a break leaving me in control (under the supervision of the midwife in charge). The lady then asked for a top-up of her epidural, which I couldn't do on my own so I went and found a midwife to do it for me. As she was giving the top-up, the baby's heartbeat dropped. Just at that moment the midwife in charge popped her head around the door and we called her over. She immediately went and called doctor to review. Doctor came in, and the baby's heart rate was normal again, but doc examined her and she had not pro-gressed from our last VE a few hours earlier. They tried taking a blood sample from the baby's head (FBS, fetal blood sample) but failed. Plan was for her to have a Caesarean because the baby's heart rate kept dropping with her contractions. I managed to get bloods from her (yippee!) and we transferred into theatre very quickly. She was having a section within minutes of being in theatre; it surprised me how quickly it was all happening! My mentor was still on her break so another midwife came into theatre with me and supervised me whilst I scrubbed and prepared to catch the baby at section. She called the paediatrician too, because it was an emergency section we had to make sure they were there in case the baby needed any medical support at delivery. The paed arrived very quickly, and the midwife told her what had been happening. Thankfully the baby came out fine. Was rather frightening though . . . And that was the beginning of a rubbish shift.

After that I had a break for an hour and then started working with another midwife, helping her care for a lady expecting twins (thirty weeks gestation) whose membranes had ruptured and she was contracting three in ten. Helped whilst anaesthetist sited epidural and then tried to catheterise her. After saying to midwife 'Don't worry, I will do this, done it loads before', I got the wrong bloody hole and feed the catheter into her vagina (stupid) . . . midwife got another catheter which I correctly inserted, only for it to fall out whilst I was connecting the bag. Got another catheter and inserted it and it was done. Confidence now on the floor. Felt rubbish and tired (it was 7.30a.m. by now). Day staff were having handover and when they finished, an experienced midwife came in and said she was taking over (relief, can get to bed now!), then the midwife I was working with asked me to handover to the midwife taking over from us. I did my best and gave her all the details I thought I needed to. She was very stroppy, asking awkward questions and looking at me in complete disgust as I painfully stuttered my way through all this information as coherently as possible at the end of a long night shift. Obviously on a power trip, but it worked; my confidence in my ability had by now disappeared completely (stupid cow).

So, came home, concentrating so hard to stay awake on the way. Took my kids to school and am just about to go and pick them up again. Still feel like I could sleep for a century. Nights are OK, I just feel so crappy when I am doing them. On the brighter side, all three assignments are now written, I just need to go over them and perfect them, add a few references in and check reference lists. Will do that next week when I am at uni, too much to do now whilst I am on placement.

Week Nineteen

Sunday

Have finished my four weeks on delivery. Have caught nine babies, and received five from C-sections. Was my last shift yesterday with my mentor, and it was brilliant. Completely got my confidence back. My mentor let me do everything. I admitted our lady, took a history and then did a VE. She was 3cms dilated; gave her Ranitidine, Meptid and Phenergan. Showed her how to use the Entonox and stayed with her to support her. Did another VE after 4 hours, 5cm dilated, and then arranged an epidural (she wasn't coping with pain very well), tried to cannulate but failed, mentor tried and she failed too, so anaesthetist did it for us. Performed a further VE once epidural was effective; now 6cm dilated, and did an ARM (artificial rupture of membranes). Liquor had thin old meconium in it, popped her on CTG to monitor the baby. Did all the paperwork and handed her over to night staff at 9.30p.m. Didn't get a catch, but felt fabulous that I had managed everything else! Rang delivery suite this morning and she had delivered at around 2a.m. (ventouse), so wouldn't have got catch anyway. Mum and baby daughter fine.

Back to uni tomorrow. Have set myself the goal of completely finishing assignments this week. Need to start on revision for exam, which is only two months away now. Want to make sure I know everything inside out!

Week Twenty

Tuesday

Have made the biggest mistake, can't quite believe it. Have forgotten all about arranging a formative assessment with my delivery suite mentor, which should have taken place last week. How could I forget to do such an important thing? My tutor asked in lectures this morning how we had all got on, if she hadn't said anything I would have gone on totally oblivious to the fact it should have been done already. Was almost honest, and said it hadn't taken place due to it being busy on delivery etc, and rang mentor at lunchtime. She now has three days off and is back in on Saturday and Sunday, so I will have to go to the hospital for this bloody assessment during my first weekend off in a month. Can't leave it any longer, as summative assessment is planned for Tuesday and that's with tutor, community mentor and hospital mentor.

And the other girls have all managed to finish their assignments. I had already planned to finish mine on Thursday and Friday this week, but again I feel like a failure as I haven't done them yet.

On top of all that, tutors keep talking about the exam and how we should have started revising. Then there's the research critique we should have started, and have now been given the task of critiquing an aspect of postnatal care from the ward using two research studies to feed back to the group. PRESSURE! Am definitely feeling like I am being sucked under. Family life is on hold, not eating properly, fainted last week (effect of working nights) and have lots of lovely spots all over my face! And I thought doing a midwifery degree in eighteen months would be manageable . . .

I know I felt like this during my nurse training, and I was expecting it again, but just feel so helplessly out of control. Everything that is important seems to be pulling me in different directions, and I am just exhausted the whole time. Perhaps I will feel better after assignments and assessments are done next week. Bloody well hope so!

Sunday

Made my way, very resentfully, to delivery suite this morning to meet my mentor and complete my formative assessment. Typically there were a lot of women in labour with not enough midwives. I think I was just finishing my sixth cup of tea when my mentor finally staggered into the coffee room apologising profusely for having kept me waiting so long. Poor thing, it wasn't her fault. If there were enough staff rostered for the shift, then things wouldn't have been quite so bad but staffing, I had quickly learnt, always seemed to be an issue. I went and made her a coffee and she sat and dutifully completed my assessment with me. I passed! But I knew I was going to pass; she had told me on the phone she had no concerns regarding my knowledge or clinical skills. Guiltily I headed home, leaving what looked like barely-organised chaos and very tired midwives.

Week Twenty-One

Friday

Have had a fabulous week. Had my summative assessment on Tuesday with my personal tutor from uni, my community mentor and my hospital mentor. Was quite scary being the centre of attention, which I hate. But, I passed it all at level three (indirectly supervised) when I only needed a level two (directly supervised) to pass! Feel so much better now that it is over and done with.

I spent the rest of the week working on the postnatal ward. First couple of shifts were disorientating, I didn't know what needed to be done and when, which always makes me feel useless. Then today it all came together and I cared for a bay and a half of women and did it all. Postnatal mother and baby checks, obs, meds, discharges, removing catheters and venflons, it was great! My mentor took a step back and let me get on with it all, and I just asked her for help if I needed to. Think it might be the first time that I have actually felt like I'm a midwife.

Week Twenty-Four

Monday

Where does the time go? Been a while since I last wrote in my diary, reflects the continuingly frenzied time I have had. Placement on post-natal ward is now finished. Did have an exciting catch in the antenatal bay of all places! The lady had been complaining of irregular contractions but didn't really look as if anything was happening. My mentor had sent me to check the lady opposite whilst she sat and chatted to this lady. All of a sudden I could hear my mentor shouting at me to get some gloves on, quickly! I did as I was told and when I got back my mentor had her hand on the baby's head seemingly holding it there in readiness for me to catch, whilst the lady was pushing for all she was worth and making a lot of noise, and her partner was just sitting there looking shell-shocked at the drama that was unfolding right in front of him! So, the baby was delivered by *moi* in the antenatal bay (there was not a chance of getting to delivery suite – this baby had decided it was coming!). An exquisitely beautiful little girl with lashings of dark hair had made her entrance into the world. We cuddled her up in bed with her rather surprised Mum and Dad. I made my way around the other ladies in the bay, all rather pale and scared after hearing the screams and commotion of the delivery, trying to offer reassurance to them!

Have had three lovely thank-you cards and boxes of chocolates from a few of the women I have cared for . . . always nice, could get used to this! Did my first induction of labour (IOL) by performing a VE and then popping a Prostin gel into the posterior fornix (the large recess behind the cervix) of the vagina. The lady only needed the one Prostin and she went on to deliver that night. Must have put it in the right place then!

As a knock-on effect of delivery being very busy, the postnatal ward has been horrendous, full to bursting with loads to do. Ended up working on my own and just asking for help when I needed it. Not ideal but needs must, and I am sensible enough to get help if necessary. Most of the work was nursing jobs anyway, obs, meds etc. Was looking forward to a lovely day off yesterday, maybe a bit of Christmas shopping, but it wasn't to be. Was having a nice cup of tea at 8a.m. Kids still asleep, chatting to hubby and phone rang. It was theatres, where I used to work, desperate for me to do a bank shift. Couldn't say no. So off I trotted like a lamb to the slaughter. Got there by 9a.m. and they had four ladies queuing for C-sections! Was quite nerve-racking actually, preparing to be a scrub nurse for a C-section, couldn't remember what half of the instruments were called, although by the second section I was already back into the old swing of things. Was nice to work as a nurse again for the day and not be a student, although I did keep signing 'Student Midwife' instead of 'Staff Nurse'! Whoops!

Got home at about 9p.m. to find none of the washing had been done, none of the cleaning or tidying had been done, the kids' school uniforms weren't ready, their packed lunches hadn't been made, their homework hadn't been done, in fact nothing had been done. Makes me so mad. I had been at work all weekend. I did it all this morning when I should have started my revision. Have now done three hours of revision and am sick of it already! Feel like I will never remember all the names for the female reproductive organs, basic ones are easy but all the different parts, and ligaments and muscles, arggghhh! So am having a break, will carry on later. Good news is I have finally finished all three assignments, just need to print them and then hand them in.

Week Twenty-Six

Friday

STRESSED! Am stressed big time. Actually I cannot verbalise how bloody stressed I am, it's horrid. Sat mock exam at the end of last week. Anatomy and physiology (A&P) was twenty multiple choice questions and three essay questions. Got results two days later and was devastated. Essays were fine; got 70%, 75% and 75% – all 'A's. Multiple choice got 36%, a fail (40% is a pass). Have never failed anything, and had spent ALL of the previous week revising A&P so I should have been OK. (Other girls in group got 46%, 41%, 36% and 33%, and 'A's or 'B's in essays). I just think it's shite, they negatively mark these multiple choice questions. Here is an example;

'Diuresis in the immediate postnatal period is caused by:

a) decrease in oxytocin
b) decrease in plasma volume
c) falling levels of oestrogen
d) increase in progesterone
e) increase in prolactin'

The correct answers are apparently b, c and e (although I would argue that e was not involved in diuresis but the uni have said it is, and what they say is final). If you circle b, c and e you get five marks (one for each correct answer circled and one for each incorrect answer left blank). If you were to circle a, b and d you would get minus three (minus one for each incorrect answer circled and each correct answer not circled and one for the correct answer circled). If it hadn't been negatively marked I would have got 60% (more like it). However, some of the questions are ambiguous, they are not black or white, right or wrong, and because you can only circle the answers there is no opportunity to explain why you have chosen them. We have two shots at this exam and if we fail, we are then kicked off the course . . . therefore I feel STRESSED! Spent the day revising with the girls, and am revising again on Monday. Feel good about revising, but guilty that husband and children have been left at home without me over Christmas. Feeling rubbish.

To add insult to injury my pager has bust, and I have missed the delivery of one of my caseload women as a result. Because it is Christmas, uni is closed and I can't get it fixed. Have been good all Christmas, not drinking and warning friends and family that I may have to leave at a moment's notice. Basically, I have been on edge, and consequently a moody mother and wife. Why an earth did I think training to be a midwife was a good idea? Feel like I should jack it all in and go back to nursing, before it's too late. Least exam is two weeks away, which gives me time for more revision . . . seems like that's all I ever do. Have just eaten half a sticky toffee pudding with half a tub of double cream. Feel sick, and am going to bed.

Week Twenty-Nine

Monday

Exam day. Have not had a life for the past couple of weeks. Have revised and revised and revised. Spent a few days with the other girls revising too. Poor hubby and kids . . . and it was right through Christmas and New Year, but I just haven't been able to focus on anything. Life has been well and truly on hold.

So, had arranged for the other girls to meet at mine at 7.20a.m. so we had plenty of time to get to uni for 9a.m. One arrived at 7.20a.m. and the other two got here at 7.45a.m. so it was pushing it to get to uni in time. We have to go along a very busy road where there are always hold-ups during the rush hour on the way into the city. Within minutes of getting onto dual carriageway, we had stopped in the fast lane, traffic chocka in front of us. Rang hubby who looked on Trafficmaster, big crash en route. CRAP! All traffic diverting the only other way we know. Sat in traffic for forty-five minutes. Had drunk four cups of tea before leaving, so at this point I was trying really hard not to pee myself in the back of the car. Was now 8.30a.m. Close to a motel, had to stop and pee. Other student midwife rang; she was at uni wanting to know where we all were. Explained; she said she would let tutor know. Traffic cleared, foot to the floor for all of two minutes, then more hold-ups, traffic stopped ahead again. All chain-smoking like mad. Now 8.52a.m. No way on earth we were going to get to uni for 9a.m. Rang other student midwife to ask her to tell tutor. Tutor was there with her. Explained to tutor, who said exam starting at 9.30a.m. and that we could enter up to thirty minutes into exam but wouldn't be given extra time at the end. DOUBLE CRAP! Still all chain-smoking. Silence in car. Traffic clearing. Foot to floor again. Get to uni at 9.20a.m. (God knows how). No parking spaces . . . there are always parking spaces . . . find a nice spot of open grass and dump car. All run to pee (again). Other student had got us all a cup of tea, bless her. Tutor comes to take us to exam room.

Heart beating loudly. Walk to exam room. Trying hard not to scream and run away. Room is very hot . . . Too hot. Sit at the back in the corner. Hands shaking, spill tea all over paper! Ooops! (Least I hadn't written on it at that point!) Hee hee hee! First section, the dreaded multiple choice paper, have thirty minutes. Just as bad as I had expected, definitely knew some answers, had to try and work out the others through a process of elimination, was over already. Next part was sections two, three and four; all essay questions, fifty minutes allotted to each section. Antenatal was choice between screening tests for fetal anomalies and Down's or minor disorders of pregnancy. Did minor disorders. Intrapartum was choice between pain relief in early labour, information-giving and facilitating choice or monitoring normal progress in first stage and supporting woman. Did pain relief. Postnatal was care of the perineum after a second degree tear and reducing risk of genital tract sepsis or physiological jaundice of the neonate, midwifery management and supporting the mother. Did jaundice. Finished exam with a stinking headache and the urgent need to pee (yet again!).

Next couple of hours are still a blur. We all had lunch in Tesco. Smoked a lot (again) in the car on the way back to mine. Had lots of cups of tea and discussed multiple choice paper, managing between us to remember all the questions and answers which I have typed up so we can try and work out how well we did (not sure if that is a good thing or a very bad thing to do!). Added up my totals and with the answers I am definitely sure of and giving myself the most negative marks possible for the answers I am not sure of, I think I will have a minimum of 48%, which thankfully is a pass. The other girls are very worried because they remember answering a lot of the questions incorrectly, but I will help them work out what they got at uni tomorrow. So, to celebrate getting through it without having a complete nervous breakdown, I am cooking a king prawn vindaloo for tea . . . yummy!

Feel like I can move on now and focus on the next essay, due in three months. Sounds like a long time, but it's the research critique which I know is going to be really hard, so want to try and get it started soon to give myself the best possible chance. As well as that I have to put in my integrated study proposal (dissertation proposal), which involves choosing a topic and collecting the main pieces of research to be critiqued and arranging a meeting with my tutor to discuss it, lots of work really. Never mind. Just keep thinking it is all going to be worth it when I qualify. It's the best job in the world!

Friday

Am so glad this week is over. We were told today to expect the results from our essays in six weeks, and the results from our exam in eight weeks . . . Seems like forever to wait, but hey. Had a session on putting together our proposal for our dissertation first thing, followed by a lecture on the care of the preterm neonate. With ten minutes to go I had to ask the lecturer if it was OK for me to make a quick exit at midday because I had booked my next session for my tattoo removal for 12.15p.m. Made it there in time; she used a different laser today, which hurt . . . a lot! Made it back to uni in time for the afternoon session on fetal skull birth injuries. We were given a model fetal skull by the rather dippy lecturer (bless her, she tries her best). After an hour of her mumbling, um'ing and arr'ing we were all bored. The girls next to me were playing noughts and crosses. I decided to modify my fetal skull by giving it luminous eyes (from a chocolate bar wrapper), taking a photo of it and Bluetoothing it to the other girls, which resulted in us all laughing hysterically. The lecturer just carried on seemingly oblivious to it. Bizarre!

Managed to prepare a presentation on Potter's Syndrome and Congenital Hip Dysplasia yesterday, meaning I can relax for the weekend. My daughter's having a birthday party tomorrow so that will keep me busy. Although after discussing the dissertation this morning, I may start reading through all the information I have collated on birth plans (the focus of my dissertation), so I can pick out my key texts. Must remember to email my personal tutor too, I need to arrange a meeting with her to discuss my chosen focus but she can be difficult to pin down (and that's putting it mildly).

Sunday

Lovely weekend, apart from lack of sleep due to my tattoo blistering and being extremely painful! Had settled children in bed and had a shower and was nice and chilled on the sofa, ready for a lazy evening of TV with a glass of red wine poured and ready when my mobile rings, unknown number, answered it and it was a midwife calling from delivery suite. One of my caseload ladies had been admitted and was 4cm dilated, could I make my way in? OF COURSE I COULD!!! Still had wet hair from shower . . . ran upstairs to get dressed, and put a little make-up on (an attempt to make myself look human). Arrived within twenty minutes, she was having strong, regular contractions (three in ten) and was coping without pain relief. Her sister was there, supporting her. Took handover from the midwife, and started work. Talked about pain relief options, what positions she wanted to be in, what position she wanted to deliver in, whether she wanted an active or physiological third stage and whether the baby was to have vitamin K. Night staff came on at 9.30p.m. and I brought the oncoming midwife up to date with what was happening. She had another lady to look after and left me to it.

My lady laboured like a trooper, and was doing so well. She eventually asked for Entonox to take the edge off the pain, and this worked really well for her. At 11.45p.m. I did a VE and she was 8cm dilated, with bulging membranes. Within an hour she was involuntarily pushing, her waters had broken. She was now squatting and kneeling, holding the bed for support and I called my mentor back into the room. Baby's head began to become visible and I opened my delivery set and got my gloves on ready to catch! It was quite difficult seeing what was going on because of her position, but she was comfy, so I ended up sitting, kneeling – almost lying – on the floor to get a good view of the baby's progress. Baby's head was delivered, followed quickly by her body. I was all fingers and thumbs trying to keep the baby off the floor and Mum sat backwards propped against my mentor, whilst I dried the baby and held her up to Mum for her first cuddle. I clamped the cord and her sister cut the cord whilst I popped the Syntometrine injection in Mum's leg (for active third stage). After about five minutes I delivered the placenta. It was a relaxed delivery, how it was meant to be; we all sat there for a while and marvelled at what had just taken place, smiles all round!

I wrapped the baby, and gave her to the sister for a cuddle whilst we helped Mum onto the bed. I went and got tea and toast for her and took the placenta away to check; it was complete with ragged membranes. I returned to the room to weigh the baby, do check and give vitamin K, and then completed notes whilst mentor kept a close eye on what I was doing. By the time Mum had had a shower, and all the paperwork was completed, it was 3a.m. and I headed home, tired but very happy. Got to bed at 3.30a.m. knowing that only three hours later I would be getting up and heading to uni for a day of lectures.

Week Thirty

Wednesday

Got home from uni yesterday and collected kids from after school club to be told that my son was being excluded because of his behaviour. BOMB SHELL. Came home numb. No club means no midwifery course for me. Talked for hours with hubby about possible options, and there are none. Son is most important thing and need to get him sorted, even if that means that I have to sacrifice my course. Went to bed, and couldn't stop crying. Got up this morning, still feeling numb, very tearful too. Took them to school and the manager of the club came over to me in the playground for a chat. I told her that I would quit my course, and she seemed to change her mind, saying that they could put him on trial for a couple of weeks and see how things go. Terrible timing; I explained to her that he was having a behavioural assessment (arranged by myself) at school in two weeks' time, and I was hoping for some input on how to handle his behaviour and help him. When I got home I rang the school nurse, and have arranged for her to come and see me next week. She said she could do some sessions with him at school focusing on how he handles anger, and building on promoting socially acceptable behaviour ... sounds promising.

My mum came over and we talked things through. She doesn't want me to quit. Just feel like this is all too much hassle, juggling uni, placements, essays, kids, feel worn out. Am again considering ringing my old work and discussing whether it would be possible to go back, perhaps for two days a week so I don't lose my nursing registration, but can be at home more. Don't know what to do for the best really. Is going to take a lot of thinking through. In a weird way I don't feel that unhappy about the prospect of having to stop the course, it's almost like I have accepted that it is inevitable. The thought of not having to write millions of essays and having my life back is a good one.

Week Thirty-one

Tuesday

What a difference a week makes! My little boy has been so much easier to handle these last few days. He has been good at club . . . yippee! After a lot of indecision, I asked my sister-in-law if she would pick the kids up from school in the afternoons on the days I was working, and she has agreed. So the plan is to continue using the club before school and she will have them after school. Only time will tell . . .

Week Thirty-two

Wednesday

OMG . . . have worked so much in the last week. Did my first three shifts on SCBU (special care baby unit) last week. They are all lovely people, very welcoming and keen to share their knowledge, but it is sooo boring. It really isn't the job that I want to do, spending a twelve and a half hour shift there is like a prison sentence and I still have another four and a half weeks to go. I know I should think about it positively – I have learnt a lot already. Also did two bank shifts (both nights) in theatres where I used to work. Was so lovely to be back there, I really loved that job. We were kept busy with four C-sections and a couple of tears that needed repair in theatre. Wondered why I had ever left . . . until I drove the thirty miles home in rush-hour traffic on the motorway after being awake for twenty-four hours.

Have started the dreaded research critique assignment! Hate research, loathe it, don't get it, weird language – just pants really. Has taken me months to track down a research study to critique, was feeling brave and am going for a quantitative study as everyone says they are easier.

Still bloody hard if you ask me; all I have done so far is the introduction and critiqued the title of the study and that took me two days! Instead of doing it this morning, so far I have done two lots of washing, cleaned the bathroom, bought some books online, done the washing-up and generally tidied the house . . . hee hee hee! Must crack on and get some done, otherwise I will spend the evening feeling guilty that I haven't done any.

Friday

9.30a.m.

Have a terrible cold. Was hoping that I would be sent home from the delights of SCBU yesterday because every time I tried to do something my nose would start running and I had to stop and blow my nose, and then wash my hands, and then blow my nose and then wash my hands (get the idea?). Surely that's an infection risk, me having a heavy cold, but no, sister said that if she sent home all her staff that had a cold then she wouldn't have any staff left . . . great! Anyway, still have a cold, and am generally feeling sorry for myself because of it. Sent a text to the girls (my fellow student madwives; we have decided we must be mad to be on this course!) first thing because I was sure that one of the lecturers had told us that today was the earliest we may possibly get the results for the essays we handed in six weeks ago. None of them knew for sure so I rang the university to ask – no reply from exams office, typical. If it is anything like the nursing course I did with the same university then the results would be going onto the online message board at twelve midday. Will have to check later.

Have tried doing a bit more of my research critique, but what with this cold and worrying about results, I can't concentrate. Will text fellow student midwife and see if she fancies a break from essay and cup of tea instead. Yes, she does, am off for a natter.

1p.m.

Just got back from having a natter, and lots of cups of tea and cake! Popped computer on to carry on with essay and thought I would have a quick look at uni message board just in case the results have been published today. They are there . . . the results have been online since midday. A wonderful example of how crap the organisation is at uni. Anyway, panic over, my results are as follows:

Community Profile – 2000 words = 75%
Care Analysis – 1500 words = 74%
Reflection – 1000 words = 74%
Result = 74%

Bloody hell, I got 'A's! Yippeeeee!!! Not sure what the last result is for, or whether it is an average of the others, but I am on track for getting a first (degree). Well, maybe that's wishful thinking, but haven't written at level three before and to get 'A's is a real confidence boost. Text others to let them know results were online (in case they hadn't checked). And then rang hubby, Mum, Nan, text bro and friends, am so proud! Hopefully, results from exam, which are due in three weeks, will be just as good! Will celebrate with a bottle of red tonight I think. Working on SCBU tomorrow, but due to the fact I don't have to use my brain, I don't think having a hangover will make a blind bit of difference.

Sunday

Have finished my second week on SCBU. Am literally counting down the hours, minutes, well, seconds come to think of it. Did a twelve and a half hour shift yesterday. Was given four babies to care for with my mentor. Three of the babies had their mums there doing everything for them. The other baby's parents were there for the majority of the day, so I only had to feed him first thing. So, my long shift, all twelve and a half hours of it consisted of . . . (drum roll . . .) . . . wait for it . . . passing a nasogastric (NG) tube and tube-feeding twice, oh, and handing over one baby at the end of the shift.

Kids are on half-term this week. I managed to swap my reading week around so that I have half-term off too, just have to go to uni for lectures on Tuesday. Could really have done with using the reading week to finish the research essay, but for childcare reasons needed to do the swap. So, it means I will have to do as much of the essay in the evenings as possible, because I also have others to get on with once this one is finished.

Took the kids to the local wildlife centre for an hour today. Thought it would be a good idea to buy an annual subscription because it is so close by. Had fun wondering around watching the monkeys, tigers, meerkats . . . decided I would like to be reincarnated as a sloth. I love sleeping, think that life would suit me perfectly. God, if you are listening, sloth next time please!

Have got to prepare for our neonatal presentation, which is in a couple of weeks at uni. Have already been on various websites and requested information and leaflets from them, but now need to collate the information and compile the presentation. Think I will make a start on it tonight.

Week Thirty-three

Monday

Have had a midwifery-free day! Had a wonderful lay-in this morning, finally getting up at about 9.30a.m. to have a shower. Kids were just as lazy. Had to bribe them with chocolate to get them dressed in the end. Popped to DIY shop to get some paint and then we spent the afternoon painting the ceiling in the kitchen/dining room. Was really good fun, you should have seen us when we had finished, with splodges of paint in our hair, on our clothes and all over the kitchen – took ages to clean up!

Just got kids to bed, and have to do some midwifery stuff now. Have a meeting with my personal tutor after lectures tomorrow, so need to get my research critique printed in case she asks to look at it. Also have to try and decide on a focus for my dissertation. It's going to be about birth plans in some way or another, but have a lot more to do before I can present the proposal. Will keep me busy for a few hours tonight anyway.

Tuesday

Oh, how quickly life can become stressed again. Uni today. Had to drop kids off at brother's house (because it's half-term), so left at 7.15a.m. with kids in tow. Dropped them off, met fellow midwife I share lifts with and drove to uni, arriving at 9.10a.m. after sitting stationary on the motorway for what seemed like a week. Lectures were very dry, spent the day drawing doodles on the handouts. Felt a little uncomfortable around the others too after the results last week. We talked about it a bit, and they are disappointed at only getting 'B's and 'C's. Anyway, had to meet tutor to update her on dissertation proposal and research critique. Went OK but didn't leave her office till gone 5p.m. Then fellow midwife needed a poo, so left uni around 5.30p.m. in the end, on the way back to my brother's. Traffic . . . aaarrrggghhh, makes me so mad, sat in traffic for another hour and finally got kids at gone 6.30p.m. Hubby was working away otherwise he would have picked them up earlier. Drove home promising them fish and chips from the chippy, but pulled up outside said chippy only to find they were closed on Tuesdays. Got home at 7p.m. and made pancakes for us all.

Kids now in bed and I am all in a panic. Need to put a lot of work into dissertation proposal. Tutor not entirely happy with it. Only time we could meet over the next two weeks is tomorrow, so have to do it all tonight. Great, am feeling absolutely exhausted after such a long day, really need to sit and chill for a bit, but instead I have to stay focused and work on my proposal.

Wednesday

Was up till midnight working on my dissertation proposal, got up early and have been at it again this morning. Daughter has now gone to a birthday party and have promised son lunch out, then have to meet tutor at hospital at 1p.m.

Just got back. Tutor phoned (whilst I was driving to the hospital to meet her), and cancelled meeting, she needed to go back to uni for something she had forgotten. All that bloody work I did! Felt like screaming at her. Felt like telling her exactly how much work I had put into my proposal since yesterday at *her* request because today was the only day *she* could meet. Felt like telling her how tired I was. Felt like using a few rather explicit words . . . Could feel my heart pumping and was so angry. Took some deep breaths and tried to keep it together. I was driving past the local cinema, so decided to take my son to watch a film – it was actually rather good! Got home three hours later and emailed my proposal to my tutor. She rang me straightaway (apparently she had been waiting for it all afternoon. Tough tits!!). She is a lot happier with the concept and themes I have put together . . . sigh of relief.

Still needs a few more references, but will worry about that another time. This is supposed to be my week off. Am on strike, no more essays till next week!

Friday

Took kids to Mum's yesterday, and came back today. Was lovely. She lives in Norfolk, so we spent time by the sea which was great . . . very cold . . . but great. Kids tried crabbing but didn't catch anything. We pottered about, wandering around the little boutique shops, so relaxing. Had proper seaside fish and chips too.

Back at home now. Plan to catch up on washing, housework and clean the car tomorrow. Back to work on SCBU (oh joy) on Sunday, will be taking my essays with me to work on. Can't stand another twelve and a half hour shift sitting on my jacksy, doing bugger all!

Week Thirty-four

Monday

Feel really guilty now; after being mean about SCBU I have actually had a couple of really lovely shifts. Yesterday and today have been a little more interesting, caring for three babies who needed hourly attention helped the shift pass quicker. Popped to delivery suite yesterday and spent time chatting to the midwives, and caught up with all their news, just to remind myself that I am actually a student midwife and not a student SCBU nurse. Worked an early today and was home by 4p.m. so have just made tea, am going to pop upstairs for a bath, and then try and crack on with this research essay. Have booked to have my roots done tomorrow morning, so feel as if I should at least try and make an effort to do some tonight. Working in the community on Wednesday, and then have Thursday and Friday to really try and get the first draft done. Will keep you posted!

Wednesday

Kind of had a fabulous day. Was in the community doing an antenatal clinic. My mentor was on holiday, so worked with another really lovely (very senior) midwife. She let me get on and do everything, which was great, so took some blood, something that always frightens me, even now. Also had a woman who was a week overdue, and she agreed to have a stretch and sweep. This is where the midwife does a VE but additionally tries to insert her finger through the opening of the cervix, stretching it, in an attempt to stimulate hormone production and release, which may initiate labour. I did it! Not done one before, so again was quite nervous, but acted professionally . . . got on with it (with mentor standing with me), found cervix straightaway, got finger in easily, had a good sweep and all done. Fingers crossed the woman will go into labour soon, bless her, being a week overdue she was rather fed-up (remember the feeling well).

Anyway, this lovely (but very senior) midwife was chatting about a newly qualified midwife who has just started out in the community. Apparently lots of the women have been complaining about her because she comes across very indecisive, lacking confidence etc. so there are general concerns about her abilities. We then started talking about when I qualify and she said that the people in the know monitor students' progress and make jobs available when the ones they want qualify. So, when I qualify, if they don't make a job available I will know that they don't want me and that I don't fit in! Great!

Feeling quite apprehensive about the whole thing now. As a newly qualified midwife, I would hope that I would get support as and when I need it, but it looks like they are just chucked into working independently in the community, with no real back-up, and told to get on with it. Maybe she is just a bit of a drip. This midwife I was working with kept telling me how fantastic I was, and how good I was going to be – but she was hardly going to tell me I am rubbish is she?

Got home in time to pick kids up from school. They had had a Victorian day at school today and were both dressed in costume, bless them. My little lad had two milk teeth out at the dentist yesterday, and is still feeling quite delicate, so we enjoyed a cuddle on the sofa for ages when we got home.

Have just finished my loss and bereavement presentation . . . thought I would check my emails quickly. There was one there from my cohort leader informing us that our exam results are going to be posted online at 12.30 this Friday! SHIT! Wish in a way I didn't know that, am going to be worried sick all day tomorrow now, and all Friday morning.

Thursday

Have woken up with a horrible sore throat, am sure I keep getting poorly because I have given up smoking. Never used to get so many colds and sore throats. Dropped kids off at school and drove to meet my caseload lady that I delivered a month ago. Was so lovely to see her, and the baby. We sat and chatted, and she told me how wonderful the experience had been for her and how she was pleased that she had managed a vaginal delivery (her last baby was born by emergency lower segment Caesarean section for breech presentation six years ago). Really boosted my confidence listening to how she felt she had such a good labour. She did all the hard work, but I hope in some way I had contributed to the good experience too!

Plan for today; check presentation that I finished last night, just to make sure it is good enough, then try and do some of the research critique, can't put it off forever. Will feel sooo much better when it is done!

Friday

Have woken up with what feels like flu. Haven't had flu before, but am sure this is what it must feel like. I didn't get much sleep last night, alternated between a blocked then runny nose, horrible cough, and kept swinging from being very hot and sweaty to freezing cold. My skin hurts all over, weird . . . just feels really sensitive to touch, and am now freezing cold, even though heating is on full, and I have two jumpers and a scarf on! Think I might have to phone in sick for the weekend if it doesn't clear up. Did manage to pop to chemist this morning and have bought some cough medicine, throat lozenges, Lemsips and Ribena! Love warm Ribena when I am poorly!

So, yesterday, I managed to get quite a lot of my critique done, about a third I would say, to the point where I am happy with it and it doesn't need re-writing, and all the references are in correctly. Haven't actually managed to do any yet this morning though, but I am poorly, it is exam results day, and the clock is going so slowly. Invited one of the girls over to check her results with me because she doesn't have Internet access at home. Really hate being with someone when getting results, selfish I know, but I like to come to terms with whatever I got by myself before sharing it with others. Just hope and pray we both pass, would be awful for one of us to pass and the other one to fail. In fact, I hope all five of us pass . . . couldn't bear to think of any of us having to re-sit the bloody thing. Anyway, nothing I can do at the moment. It's now 10.40 and results are posted at 12.30. Arrrggghhh!

11.24a.m.

Have got the shakes violently, not nerves (although am obviously petrified). Have definitely got flu . . . Have had a further two mugs of warm Ribena and have added a blanket around my shoulders but my fingers are still blue. Waiting for fellow midwife to join me (have warned her I am very ill!).

3p.m.

I passed! Got 78%, an 'A', in the multiple choice paper (the one I was really worried about!), then 68% and 64%, both 'B's in antenatal and intrapartum essay sections and 50%, a 'C' in the postnatal essay section. The overall result is 60%, a 'B', apparently they don't include the multiple choice section in the overall grade, don't know why, seems unfair, but never mind. I passed! And that's the main thing. Couldn't get all excited because fellow student midwife who was with me failed. She passed two sections, but failed the other two. I tried to be supportive, but know how gutted I would feel if that had been me. We sat and chatted for a couple of hours, and she has just left to go home now. Bless her, just hope she can get through the re-sit. Will do everything I can to help her.

Anyway, now I am on my own I have just spent half an hour phoning everyone to tell them the good news. Hubby first, then Mum, Nan, Dad, and texted all my friends! Such a relief, just wish I was feeling a bit better. Off to get kids from school now, so will share the news with them too!

Saturday

Phoned in sick today. Not had a day sick yet, but feel awful. Don't know how I got kids home from school yesterday, thought I was going to pass out. Managed to get back and collapsed on sofa . . . daughter got me her duvet and I just lay there shaking. Hubby ordered pizza for tea, to celebrate my exam success, but I only managed a slice, and then went to bed. Got up at 10a.m. this morning, hubby had phoned SCBU and told them I was poorly. Feel a bit better now, took a couple of hours to get going though.

Feel guilty about having the day off sick, so have spent the afternoon wrapped in a blanket working on my dissertation proposal which needs to be presented to my tutor on Tuesday. Finally managed to put together a descent proposal on birth plans, my chosen topic. Fingers crossed she thinks it will be OK!

Sunday

Spent twelve and a half hours working on SCBU with a sister who kept calling me the student . . . enough said.

Week Thirty-five

Monday

Went into the city this morning for the next session on my tattoo . . . it hurt a lot, again. Fellow student midwife came with me (the one who failed her exam) because she wanted to pop to uni and collect her exam feedback and speak to tutors about the re-sit. Took her to a fab shop on way home for a bit of retail therapy. She didn't buy anything, I bought a winter coat. Whoops! Was better than half price, £40 instead of £85, so a bargain really.

Whilst at uni I managed to get my three essays back with the comments sheets, and my two portfolio folders which contain my life at the moment . . . everything in them has to be very carefully filled in, and I will have to work at getting them up-to-date tonight. On top of that I have the following work to plan and do:

Dissertation Proposal – due in week 36
Research Critique – 3000 words, due in week 42
Formative Clinical Assessment – due week 45
Summative Clinical Assessment – due week 47
Neonatal Care Analysis – 1500 words, due in week 49
Complex Midwifery Care Analysis – 1500 words, due in week 49
Reflection – 1000 words, due in week 49
Depressing when it's all listed like that! Had better crack on . . .

Tuesday

Spent the most depressing day ever in uni. Should have known it was going to be a bad day by the way it started. Fellow student midwife missed turning on way to uni, which put an extra thirty miles on our journey, because there was no way off the bloody motorway! So got to uni half an hour late. On the plus side, it was our last neonatal lecture. Hooray! As I said to the girls on the way there, would rather sit in a dark room sticking needles in my eyes than suffer any more neonatal rubbish. So, missed half of that lecture, had coffee for half hour then had to present dissertation proposal to lecturer. Three others went before me, took forever, and then I did mine. We all had our ideas ripped to shreds, none of us got any positive comments, in fact we all agreed at lunchtime that we should just do away with ourselves then and there. And then we had a whole afternoon of research to sit through. The word 'rubbish' just about sums up the day. Although we did have a good moan about mind-numbingly boring SCBU to lecturer who came up with some good advice. We need to arrange gynae experience at some point through the course, and she suggested that we did that during our SCBU placements, as long as we have done a minimum of 150 SCBU hours. Have just added my hours up and so far I have done ninety-one and a half hours. If I do all the shifts I am booked for I will have done 183 and a half hours . . . will do anything to not be in SCBU for one second longer than is absolutely necessary.

Fellow midwife who failed her exam is really struggling. She had the worst feedback on her proposal, and is really panicking about the exam re-sit. I have said I will do as much as I can to help her, but need to be selfish to a certain extent and concentrate on making sure I can get myself through this course, too. One of the others in the group said the same thing, when we were walking back from the library. We are all there to support each other, but we are all under a huge amount of pressure as it is.

Remembered to ring my community mentor this afternoon, and remind her that I am doing clinic with her tomorrow morning, and that I would like to spend all day with her. She said that was still OK, and we have arranged to meet at 8.30a.m. at the GP surgery to get the room ready for clinic. She is on-call tonight, and I volunteered myself to be on-call with her. There is a planned homebirth lady overdue, so fingers crossed she goes into labour tonight . . . never happens when I am on-call, so mentor has a guaranteed full night in bed ahead of her! Hee hee hee!

Two of my caseload ladies are due next week so they could go into labour at any time, so I'm making sure that my mobile is fully-charged and always within reach, just in case. Have arranged to go to a friend's for a bottle of red tomorrow night to celebrate my exam results, so what's the betting that one of them goes into labour when I am on my way there, or worse, after I have drunk half a bottle of red wine!

Thursday

Had an absolutely wonderful day with my community mentor yesterday. Clinic lasted over five hours (should have been 9a.m. till 1p.m. but was so overbooked it ended up being 8.30 till 2p.m.). Managed it all though, and caught up with some of my caseload ladies too. Then I did a booking, first one in months. We also had a few visits to do, one of which was the stretch and sweep I had done the previous week in clinic; she had delivered and I was doing a postnatal check on her and the baby, which was nice.

Today, after popping to the Post Office to send my Mother's Day pressie, and having a quick cuppa with my father-in-law (just to check he was OK), I cracked on with the proposal and got it emailed off to my tutor. She emailed me back at 2p.m. saying it was fine, and that the version she had would be submitted, so at least that's one thing out of the way! Then carried on with the research critique. Still hating every single minute of it, but got some done, so feeling a little more positive . . . just can't wait for it to be finished!

Hubby is being his usual grumpy shout-at-the-kids self. Made worse by the fact I can't work with him watching TV at top volume in the same room whilst I am trying to study. So have had to put up with a constant loud moaning and groaning, as he shouts at the kids to tidy up. If he tried tidying up with them instead of sitting on his arse things might get done quicker, without all the bad feeling. No telling him that though . . . he's always right . . . he's a man . . .

Friday

Did an early on SCBU today. When is this hell going to end? Am sure they all know how much I hate it, loathe it, would prefer to be anywhere else . . . Am now counting down the shifts and I have seven left – seven, how am I going to survive? Have tried to stay interested in what is going on, but have often found myself sitting staring at the clock daydreaming, even caught myself planning bits of my research critique, and that is rather worrying. It's hard to verbalise just how awful this whole experience is; try and think of something you love doing, something you need to practise, but love completely. Then think about instead of doing that thing that you love, being made to do something which has nothing to do with the thing that you love, for six bloody weeks. I have learnt how to pass a NG tube, and to feed using a NG tube . . . I have had it drummed into me how important it is to keep a baby warm, and encourage feeding (although I knew that already) and that's the sum total of my learning achievement. I can't wait to fill in the feedback for this block. In fact I might work out when I have completed my 150 hours and then just beg my community mentor if I can work with her for the rest of the time.

However, I would like to emphasise that the SCBU staff have been friendly, welcoming me as part of the team, and have promoted learning opportunities for me, so my dreadful experience cannot be blamed on them, although they continually slag off the midwives, knowing full well that I am a student midwife . . .

Saturday

Have lost the will to live.

Week Thirty-six

Monday

Survived my one and only night shift on SCBU. Forced myself to go . . . was thinking of excuses, but made the effort and went. When I got there, the staff were all asking how I was enjoying my placement. I tried to lie and tell them all I was having an amazing time, but I really don't think I was very convincing! One of the girls was telling me that she cried when her SCBU placement ended when she was a student nurse, couldn't hide the look of complete surprise when she said that, whoops! She went on to say that she thought I would be the same (ha bloody ha, will be crying tears of joy at never having to go back there ever ever ever again!!) Only saving grace of working a night shift is that you get a two-hour break. Should have done all nights, days are so bloody boring, could have easily slept through all of them, so actually being able to sleep away two hours of the shift was a godsend! Shock, horror . . . Have to say though that I did enjoy some of my night shift. We looked after a tiny baby (850 grams (1lb 14oz) – a twenty-nine weeker) who was on CPAP (helps with breathing but not as full-on as being ventilated). I helped change his nappy, pass an orogastric tube, reposition him etc. First time I had cared for such a wee one. Held him on the palm of my hand and it was like holding a feather.

One of my caseload ladies is due in two days' time, so am on ten-terhooks waiting for the call that she has gone into labour. Is probably going to happen at the most inconvenient time . . . like tomorrow (my little boy's ninth birthday!). All part and parcel of the course though. So, until she delivers there will be no glasses of red wine, my mobile will be with me every second of every minute of every day, I cannot venture further than say a twenty-mile radius of the hospital (so I can get there in time) . . . the joys of being a student midwife! Had better go and get dressed, sitting here at 1.30p.m. in my dressing gown and bed hair, not a good look. Have just been trying to log onto the online secondary school admissions page; applied for my daughter's school last year, and it was on the radio earlier that decision letters have been sent out, but haven't had anything through the post today . . . will have to try again tomorrow.

Hope to get more of my critique done tomorrow too, while kids are at school. Got loads done last week and feel a lot happier about the whole thing now. Probably a load of rubbish, but at least I have put something together! Once that is finished I need to write the neonatal care analysis, am going to make my focus passing a NG tube, although I am incredibly tempted to write it on 101 things I would rather be doing with my time! Then there's the reflection to write too; will probably focus this on VEs because that is a key skill and there is a lot of research out there I can utilise. By that time I will be back on midwifery placements, and can write my complex care analysis although I haven't got a clue what it's going to be based on yet! Have it all planned, just need to keep up!

Hours of boredom spent on SCBU – 122

Hours of boredom still left to endure on SCBU – 49.5 – fuck.

Tuesday

'Would you like a cup of tea?' This was the whispered wake-up call I got this morning from my little boy who is nine today, and had woken up at 6.30a.m. all excited! So, I got all his pressies together and he opened them in bed. Took an hour of gentle persuasion to then get him up and dressed; he kept telling me that all his friends have a day off from school on their birthday! Cheeky monkey! Eventually drove them both to school and it started snowing, so that made his day. Have promised to take him to Frankie and Benny's for tea – he loves it when they play Cliff Richard's song 'Congratulations'!

Have managed to load up the dishwasher and get that going, put on a load of washing, put a load of wet washing in the tumble dryer, fold up some dry washing and make a huge ironing pile (will do that later). Have also put up all little one's birthday cards, and blown up lots of balloons ready for when he comes home from school. Need to crack on with my essay. Haven't heard from caseload lady, will have to see if she is at clinic tomorrow . . .

3p.m.

Have managed to get another large chunk of my research essay finished. Just have to write the section which outlines a strategy for incorporating the findings into my area of clinical practice now . . . won't be hard seeing as I have ripped the study to shreds and won't want to apply any of their findings to practice! Hee hee hee . . . Feel a whole lot better for working on it all day. Can enjoy my little one's birthday now!

Thursday

Had another fantastic day in the community yesterday. Clinic was busy but good, apart from one poor lady whom I tried to get blood from twice and failed, leaving her with huge bruises, poor thing couldn't stop apologising. Did a couple of visits in the afternoon and a booking (a foreign lady, needed a translator, all very time-consuming but a good learning experience for me). Got home at 6.30p.m. tired, but happy that I had finally had a day that was used constructively (unlike boring SCBU). Spent an hour updating my portfolio with all the antenatal, postnatal and booking visits I had done through the day; just need to get it all signed by my mentor next time I see her.

There was a letter waiting for me at home from the school doctor. She said she was going to have another meeting with the children's mental health team, with the possibility of diagnosing a mild form of ADHD (attention deficit hyperactivity disorder). Am so relieved that someone has finally acknowledged that my little boy isn't just naughty, but that there may be some cause for his behaviour. What really makes me mad is that the school, and childminder, club etc. have not instigated anything like this before, and that my GP ignored my requests for an assessment on him earlier. Anyway, looks like we are finally heading in the right direction now.

So, plans for today: have already done the washing, loaded the dishwasher and had a general tidy-up. Little boy was very argumentative this morning, so feeling a little low . . . hate arguing with him, but he never listens and always answers back. Can see it affects my daughter too, she sits there looking all sad, and it makes me feel like such a failure. It's now 10.30a.m. and I am going to spend the next few hours on my research critique, am hoping to write the first draft of the final section . . . Just sent a text to fellow student midwife (one who failed her exam). She is with others revising for the re-sit. Felt really left out that she hadn't invited me; thought we were quite close. Have to be selfish too and think of myself and the essays I have got to write . . . but all the same.

6.10p.m.

First draft almost finished. Have had enough for one day; am going to carry on with it on Monday next week (working on SCBU tomorrow and Saturday, and taking little boy out for his birthday treat on Sunday).

Friday

Warning; you are about to enter the Twilight Zone . . . I actually had a good shift on SCBU! Shock horror. Started the day by ringing SCBU to tell them my car wouldn't start and I would be in as soon as possible. Was only a little white lie. Took kids to before school club and made my way to hospital, changed into scrubs and was on SCBU only half an hour late. Was given handover by the nurse in charge, who is really nice, and was told to float for the day and get involved in anything interesting that was happening. So I did, and it was great. The time went so quickly, it was 2p.m. and lunchtime before I knew it! Got back after lunch to find a new term baby had been admitted with low blood sugars and low temperature. After an hour, the baby was ready to go back to ward (blood sugar wasn't as bad as first thought, and temperature was now OK), so I was sent to delivery suite to get some clean clothes from Mum to dress her baby. On delivery suite all the midwives were sitting round their station, and one of them said 'Hello' and asked me how I was doing, so I had a chat with her. There were a couple of other student midwives on, and one that I didn't recognise asked how the course was going. I told her I had a couple of caseload ladies due now; she does too. She is in her third year, and has so far got twenty-four catches (we have to get forty to qualify), to which I replied that she'd better pull her finger out and hurry up ... stupid thing to say ... they have fourteen-week placements on delivery suite, and she has another six months before her course finishes so will have plenty of time to do extra shifts on delivery if needed, so that went down well. Made my excuses and got the clothes I needed from the room, but when I walked back past the midwives' station they were still all sitting there and lowered their voices as I walked past (obviously talking about me). Talk about making me feel small ... got back onto SCBU and actually felt wanted and liked.

I know midwives have the reputation of feeling that they are better than the rest and I have always aspired to be one, but making somebody feel like that is horrible. It's the ones that have been midwives for years, the 'dragons' as I like to call them, that look at you as if you are worthless that are the worst ... But, saying that, when I finished at 4p.m. I walked through delivery suite to leave and one of the very experienced midwives (not a dragon) was there. She stopped what she was doing and asked how I was and how things were going, which made me feel a little better.

Have got a full twelve and a half hour shift on SCBU to look forward to tomorrow. But with only five babies, and two staff nurses plus me hopefully it will be OK ... We'll see. From what the girls said today, the senior nurse who is on is a right lazy cow and will get me to do everything, and if I remember correctly she was the only one who made me stay till the end of the shift and hand over the baby I had been caring for.

Week Thirty-seven

Monday

Drum roll please ... 141 hours is the total number of hours I have spent on SCBU. Have to do a minimum of 150 hours, so only 9 hours to go. Hooray! OK, seriously now, I actually had a really good shift on Saturday. Nurse in charge was a lazy moo, a very nice lazy moo, but a lazy moo none the less. We had five babies on the unit; one nurse took two, another nurse took two and the nurse in charge and I had one. I actually did everything for this baby throughout the shift (apart from calculate and prepare drugs), so I was kept busy. As a novice at all this kind of stuff, a feed would take a good ten minutes to provide the nursing care, plus five minutes to chart all the observations, plus five minutes for changing a nappy if needed, so only sat on my arse for forty minutes out of every hour. Not bad for a SCBU shift!

In a funny kind of way, I will miss working on there. Although I was mortified when one of the staff nurses suggested I register with the bank to come and cover shifts for them. As a registered nurse I could work there, if I wanted to, which I DON'T! Obviously didn't say that, and tried to sound enthusiastic at the opportunity to go back. Not sure that I pulled it off though, hee hee hee!

Am going to finish my research essay today, finally. Have only got about 300 words left to write, so am not going to let myself do anything else until the awful thing is finished. Then I am going to email it to fellow student midwife (who was a research nurse for ten years) and ask her kindly to read it for me. If she trashes it, I plan on going into my back garden, digging a big hole and burying myself in it! As a master of distraction techniques I have already done a load of washing and the washing-up, had two cups of tea, and nearly bought a new sofa in the half-price sale. Got junk mail through the door, and looked online, and am very tempted, might have to have another look in a little while to see if I still like the sofa. Have a cream leather one at the mo, which is lovely, but after numerous community visits to the rather deprived housing estates I have come to view what used to be my gorgeous sofa in a different light! This one is fabric; same style, but warm fabric. Have found leather can be quite harsh in the cold weather, would be nice to have a cosy sofa, and it's only £300 – bargain!

Still no news on my caseload lady, who is now five days overdue. Really fancied a couple of glasses of red wine last night (to get over the trip to the ice-rink with the kids yesterday morning), but made myself only have a very small one in case the call came – it didn't. This isn't getting my essay done! Right, am not returning to these pages till it's finished . . .

11.30a.m

No, it's not done, have only briefly looked at it. Dog decided to have the squits, and has squitted on every carpet in the bloody house. So have had the disinfectant out, and now the house stinks of a mixture of dog poo and disinfectant . . . yuk. Then catalogue delivery arrived, little boy needed new school shoes (again, already), so just happened to order some new jeans and tops at the same time! Spent half hour trying them all on, and am now on a crash diet because they all looked hideous. Need to join the gym.

1.25p.m.

Yippee! Have finished first draft and emailed it to my tutor. Tutors can only read 10% of each essay, but have asked her to look at final section because that's the bit I am not too sure about. Am over by 150 words (that's over the 10% allowance too), always write more than am supposed to, and then it takes hours to chop out words. You would think that a 3,000 word essay, well 3,300 word essay (including extra 10%) would be plenty of words, but oh no, not for me!

House still smells of dog poo and flowery disinfectant. Yuk. Dog is now asleep under the kitchen table behind me. Am listening out for squitting sounds! Have got an hour and a half before I have to get the children from school so I am going to make a start on the neonatal care analysis now. This one is only 1500 words, am hoping that the experience will be somewhat better than the clinical placement itself! Feels good, no more research.

7.30p.m.

OK, so didn't get much of neonatal essay done . . . Wrote the intro though, and have completed a spider diagram ready to hit the library and get some research together for it. House no longer smells of poo; always a good thing. Am mega-hungry, think I will have to postpone the start of my crash diet till tomorrow, seeing as I had fish and chips for tea, and am about to have a bowl of Coco Pops! Sent text to fellow student midwife who failed exam because I offered to help her do some revision tomorrow and she hasn't got back to me yet. And still no telephone call about my caseload lady.

Tuesday

Fellow student midwife got back to me last night and I arranged to pick her up at 9.30a.m. and drive to another fellow student midwife's house to do some revision. Didn't quite work out that way! We got there and had a natter and a cup of tea, then some more natter and another cup of tea, then we wrote a list of things we need to discuss with tutor (have her tomorrow for day at uni), then another cup of tea. By this time, we were all hungry so pigged out on bacon sarnies and chocolate muffins (what crash diet?). So at about 12.30 we started work, not revision though – student midwife whose house we were at had been through a rough few days and was feeling like everything was getting too much for her (bless her, I know how that feels). She had not prepared the presentation we are giving tomorrow and was panicking . . . so we did her presentation together. Took about an hour and a half to do, but it is all finished. I needed to get home for the children, so had to leave then (still no revision done).

The drive home was about an hour, through lovely countryside, and at one point there was a huge barn owl flying along level with the car. It was so amazing; they really look beautiful when they are flying. Kids were impressed when I told them about it when I got them home from school!

Got home to a voicemail message on my mobile from uni. The tutor we are supposed to have has been off sick today and they are not sure whether she will be back tomorrow. They are going to ring me at 7.30a.m. to let me know. Rang community mentor and explained what was going on and she has said that she is happy for me to spend the day with her if uni is cancelled; I just need to turn up for clinic. Hopefully I will get the day in clinic with her because lots of my caseload ladies are booked in, and my lady who is a week over is booked for a stretch and sweep.

Just on way up to bed when I had a call from one of the three-year student midwives who I had worked with in my old job, when I was a nurse and she was an maternity care assistant (MCA). She is struggling to write her literature critique and wanted some advice. Have emailed her my nursing literature critique, which was a level one essay I got an 'A' for, so hope it helps her. We had a chat, and I told her all about SCBU. She has had a block in uni but is back on placement soon. Think she is struggling to juggle placement, uni, essays, revision, presentations and family life just like I am . . . least I only have to do it for eighteen months. Not sure how I coped doing it for three years as a student nurse, and the midwifery course seems so much more intense than the nursing.

Tried to go to bed again and my mum phoned! She has a new job (long story), which is fabulous news! So chatted with her for a good half hour. Hubby came in and asked if I had a sore ear . . . cheeky bugger . . . but then again, suppose I had been on the phone for nearly two hours by that point. Third time lucky, am off to bed now.

Wednesday

No uni, tutor sick, so am going to go to clinic this morning with my community mentor. Have just spoken to her on the phone and she sounds pleased to have some extra help in what is always a really busy clinic. Feel desperately guilty that I am not helping fellow student midwife revise. She had phoned me last night and asked if I could meet her at the garage because her car has a flat tyre, and take her into uni from there to do some revision. Did send her a text and mention about my possible clinic, and that it will mean one day less on SCBU (HALLELUJAH, hallelujah, hallelujah!). She rang me this morning after uni was cancelled and said I should go to clinic . . . feel rubbish . . . really want to help her. I've offered Friday and two days next week, just need to keep up with stuff myself too. Hey ho.

6p.m.

Am knackered. Clinic lasted till 1.30p.m. and was really good. Saw loads of my caseload ladies; the one who is a week overdue was there. I did a stretch and sweep so am hoping that gets things going for her. Then I did a booking (another one with an interpreter), before heading back to the surgery to meet up with another one of my caseload ladies. Ended up helping in that clinic too, volunteering to go in and help next week. It is the preceptorship midwife who will be doing next week's clinic, the one who qualified a few months ago, and everyone is moaning about how rubbish she is. She's just slow at everything and constantly questioning herself – hope I don't end up like that. When I offered my services to the team leader she said she thought I would do a better job of the clinic on my own! Boosted my confidence anyway! So I will be going in when I am on annual leave to help her.

Am doing a long day on SCBU tomorrow. Have the joy of telling them that I will not be there on Friday because I worked today! Will put Friday down as a study day instead. SCBU hours are reducing by the minute! Hooray!!!

Had better ring fellow student midwife and see how she got on today with her revision. Still feeling guilty but really needed to get some more clinic experience.

Thursday

Had fantastic shift on SCBU. Really felt like I was useful today. There were nine babies, eight of which were on hourly feeds; two were very poorly and fitting quite regularly, one was very small and still on CPAP. I was allocated the care of three hourly-fed babies with my mentor, and I helped with the other babies too. Just felt like it all clicked suddenly, and I was helpful instead of just getting in the way. Was able to find things in the storeroom, use the blood gas machine independently and generally be useful!

Kept popping back and forth to delivery suite in case any of my ladies were admitted. One of them was, but it was a false alarm and she was sent home again. Saw one of the midwives I worked with whilst on my delivery suite placement and she asked when I was going back there. I told her and she said she would put her name down to work with me again . . . that was nice, made me feel wanted and liked!

Found out via one of the paediatric consultants that my triplet caseload lady delivered by emergency section a couple of days ago at another hospital, so that's one more crossed off my list . . . Poo. Have just got home after twelve and a half hours, happy but tired.

Friday

Plan was to help fellow student midwife revise today so I met her at uni in the library at 10a.m. By 10.30 we had drunk a cup of tea and I had printed all the bits I needed for my neonatal essay. We then got our diaries out and tried to sort out a few days of revision over the next few weeks; when I could do it she couldn't and when she could do it I couldn't, so we have left it that we might do a few evenings and definitely the weekend before the exam. We shall see . . . So, we then had a look at a few exam questions together and talked them through. At midday we decided to pop out for some lunch, and just happened to pass DFS on our way and the urge to look at the sofa I liked was too great. I didn't like the sofa I had been looking at, but did like another one that was more than twice the price. Bought it . . . deserve it after putting up with being on SCBU for so long.

Back to village and to kids' school for an assembly where daughter was getting an achievement certificate. Really hot now, so after school we came home and dumped all the bags in the house and took our little doggie for a lovely walk over the fields in the sunshine . . . felt like summer was on the way.

Saturday

Just got back from my last day on SCBU! There is a God . . . It was very busy with lots to do so time just whizzed past. I had taken some chocolates in as a thank-you pressie for the girls, and we ate them . . . all! They still want me to join the bank and go back to cover shift when they are short of staff, but there is nothing on this earth that would make me want to do that (hee hee hee!). Was a bit peeved when I popped to delivery suite to get something . . . I had a quick look in the delivery book and one of my caseload ladies came in and delivered yesterday morning. They didn't phone me, and when I went to the postnatal ward to see her she said she had asked them to call me so I could be there with her. I don't think the delivery suite mid-wives realise what a lot of work goes into caseloading women. We have to book them at the beginning of their pregnancy, and see them as often as possible through their antenatal clinic appointments, all takes a lot of organising to make sure we meet all of the criteria in our portfolios. Was so angry that my shyness dissipated; I had a good old moan to one of the dragon midwives who just happened to be in charge on delivery suite and she promised to make sure it was handed over to all staff that students need to be called. Won't hold my breath . . . SCBU didn't let me leave early, so have worked a full twelve and a half hours, with only a half-hour break. Just got home and it's now 9.45p.m. I can't wait to get to bed . . .

Phone just rang. Was delivery suite. One of my ladies (the one who is really overdue and I gave a stretch and sweep to on Wednesday) is in labour and they are ringing to let me know! Bloody typical . . . can't really say no now, can I? Not after having a whinge earlier! She's a first time mum too, so could be a long night.

Sunday

5p.m.

Was a long night! Got to delivery suite at 10p.m. My lady was being looked after by the midwife who delivered my other caseload lady the day before without calling me. Felt a bit awkward; wasn't sure if she was only ringing me because of my moan earlier, and not because she wanted to, but anyway . . . The look on my lady's face when I went into the room was wonderful. She looked so pleased to see me, and she gave me a huge hug! Her hubby was there too. I started all the intrapartum notes, labelling them up and taking baseline obs whilst we chatted. She was on the birthing ball and using Entonox to good effect. She was 4-5cm dilated. She told me how she had been in labour since I had done a stretch and sweep last Wednesday. She had been into delivery suite three times since then thinking it was starting, but it was just a long latent phase . . . So she was knackered, not had much sleep at all, and was completely fed up by this point.

After a few hours she requested stronger pain relief, so I did another VE to assess her progress. She was 5cm dilated. She decided to have some Meptid (an opioid analgesic), given by intramuscular (IM) injection. So my mentor and I went to get it for her. When we got back she had changed her mind. She wanted to carry on with the Entonox and see how she went. Another couple of hours later her contractions had slowed down, to the point of almost stopping. She was very tired. Spoke to midwife in charge and we decided to offer her an ARM (artificial rupture of membranes), this can help kick-start labour again, and she agreed. So I performed an ARM, she was still 5cm dilated at this point. The plan now was to reassess in two hours. Two hours later, she was progressing slowly. Contractions still not frequent enough, or strong enough. Next step, IV augmentation, so up goes the drip, on goes the CTG. Within minutes we see a deep early deceleration (the baby's heart rate dropped lower than normal); this continued for the next few contractions so we call the midwife in charge, who in turn requests an obstetric view. Outcome being that all is OK and that we should continue with drip (IV Synto) for the time being, observing the CTG carefully. By about 7.30a.m. my poor lady was ready to collapse, she was so tired. My mentor talked to her about having an epidural and she agreed. By 8a.m. it was sited and working and she was getting some well-earned sleep. Morning staff had come on, and because I had just worked twenty-two and a half hours out of the last twenty-four, I couldn't stay any longer. I said my goodbyes and came home . . . Now I really did need my bed!

I woke up at midday and had a lovely lunch with kids. It had been raining hard all through the night and it was still coming down with no let-up. The river running through our village had burst its bank, and hubby, kids and dog went for a walk to have a look while I settled into the bath. Rang delivery suite to check on my lady's progress – she had an emergency section two hours after I had gone, for failure to progress and an oedematous cervix (where the cervix swells and acts as a barrier stopping the baby's head from descending). Asked midwife to let her know that I would pop in tomorrow to see her and the baby.

Have been through rather a roller coaster of emotions yet again over the last twenty-four hours. From complete and utter joy at not having to go back to SCBU, to a real downer when I found out one of my ladies had delivered and I wasn't called, to paranoia that they didn't ring me because they don't like me (I am the weird student, or the odd one that they all bitch about), to a boost in confidence when I independently cared for my labouring woman for most of the night, to sheer exhaustion from being awake for so long, to guilt for not being at home with my kids . . . This is what it is really like being a student midwife.

After my bath I had a cleaning urge because the whole house was so filthy, obviously hubby hadn't attempted to lift a finger and actually do any housework or washing. Started with the living room, moved on to kids' bedrooms and bathroom. Did kitchen, and then started on the mountain of washing. Realised that I love my sofa, so rang sofa people and cancelled the one I had ordered. Fickle, I know . . . Kids don't break up for Easter till Thursday, so have four days to write my neonatal care analysis and finish off my research critique. Supposed to be on annual leave, but if I have a proper break it would be a mad rush to get all these essays done, so don't have any choice but to use the time studying. Roll on Christmas when I qualify – hopefully!

Week Thirty-nine

Monday

Am having a day off! Well, nearly. I popped into town and opened bank accounts for my kids. Thought I had better, that way I can pop a bit in every month and help them start to save for uni or a car etc. Long way off, but good to start too early rather than too late. Then bought my favourite perfume, 'Lovely' by Sarah Jessica Parker. Love it, love it, love it! Also bought some wonder face cream that is the only one that is meant to work. Will keep you posted (cost £17 so had better bloody work!). Then bought a couple of new cushions for my sofa I am now keeping (!) and some photo frames for the family photos we had professionally taken back at Christmas time, and some little notebooks, handy for having in my pocket to write bits in when on placement. Next I bought a new pair of black trousers for placement, as my arse has grown too big for the ones I've got!

After my little shopping spree I headed for the hospital to see my lady from Saturday night. Got onto postnatal ward and my hospital mentor was there, we sat and had a chat for a little while and she updated me on all the gossip. Showed her my wonder cream and she took a before photo, when I see her again it will be in about a month so then we can compare and see if it works! Found my lady and sat and had a chat with her for a bit and a cuddle with her little baby. Gutted I missed the delivery . . .

Now I am back home, I have cleaned the house (yet again), put my new cushions on the sofa (fabulous!), put photos in the new frames and put them up on the wall in the living room, done loads of washing and now I am going to ring the gym to join (definitely fatter now I have stopped smoking and I hate my body, something has to be done!). My friend from when I was a student nurse has agreed to be my gym buddy, that way we can make each other go. Well, that's the idea anyway.

Just pondering something. How come I can sit here and quite happily type a page of my diary within a minute or two, but when I try and write an essay, a page takes me a week?

Tuesday

Made the final changes to my research essay this morning, making sure I changed the bits my tutor had commented on. Checked the references too and all looks good. Am 200 words over the 3,300 limit so will have to chop some out. Am going to attempt that in a mo . . .

Spent the whole afternoon trying to sort out my elective placement. It's two weeks in July where we have to go somewhere out of area and experience midwifery in a different setting. Rang some birth centres but they don't have students; rang some independent midwives but they said many of their women refuse students (so no point in doing it). Rang a famous midwife called Mary; she was lovely and said she would have loved to have had me with her but she is waiting on an operation at the moment and out of action for a while. She gave me the contact numbers of some other independent midwives, but they live too far away. Think I'm going to try and get in to a hospital close to family down south.

Got round to ringing the gym today. Have arranged to go in and join tomorrow after clinic. Have just got to buy some gym clothes and trainers so I look the part! Kids have been playing up these last few days. They constantly argue and I have had enough of it. It's only 7p.m. but they are both in bed now! Well, they will learn.

Wednesday

Had a fantastic clinic this morning. The newly qualified midwife I worked with was fabulous, and very confident in her abilities; she also had a lovely manner with the women. Don't know what the senior ones have been moaning about. We had a lovely time, chatting away and the clinic was over before I knew it!

Been home for about half an hour and just had a sandwich, was so hungry! Should be on my way to the gym to join . . . not going to happen today. Just got a phone call from delivery suite saying one of my caseload ladies is there. Her waters had broken twenty-four hours ago and she has opted to have her labour augmented. I am meant to be getting kids from school so have phoned hubby who will be home by 4.30p.m. and then I will make my way in. Just going to phone them back now and let them know that's what the plan is. Sounds stupid but am really nervous about ringing them; some midwives can be so nice and others give me the impression I will never be good enough, but anyway, am postponing the inevitable, must ring them back. It's engaged . . . frustrating! Just thought if they start a Synto drip, things could really crack on quickly, wonder how many centimetres dilated she is . . . will have to ask when I can get through. Hope I don't miss it! Knowing my luck it will be another all-nighter! Update; spoke to lovely midwife who is looking after my lady. She is 3cms dilated, she had a VE so they are committed to delivering her now. Plan is to start Syntocinon drip at 4p.m. I have said I will be there between 4.30 and 5p.m. Thankfully midwife has said that is OK, and she will call me if things hot up before then. How exciting . . . hopefully I will be getting delivery number thirteeen before the night is out!

3p.m.

Am like a cat on hot bricks; can't concentrate on anything. Have to pick up kids from school at quarter past, so am sure they will keep me busy till hubby gets home . . .

4p.m.

Got kids from school. Home now. Bag ready to grab and run out of the door as soon as hubby home. Sounds awful but can't wait till these five caseloads are done and dusted. I know I will still have the pressure of getting forty deliveries but at least I won't be on-call permanently. Have missed the odd glass of red wine every now and then!

Put make-up on in an attempt to hide my spots. Put concealer in my bag ready to hide the bags that will appear under my eyes if this turns into an all-nighter. Lip-gloss in bag too, a must for any occasion! Oh, and have put a curry pot noodle in bag for tea, and three breakfast bars to snack on too . . . no wonder I am piling on the pounds. Really should make the effort to join the gym tomorrow.

Thursday

Don't know where to start really. I feel like I have every emotion possible all at the same time, it's like they are all in a blender being churned up together. This is what happened . . .

Got to delivery suite at around 5p.m. My lady wasn't doing much but augmentation by IV infusion was due to be started. By the time we had got it set up, it was 6p.m. and off we went. Contractions started almost immediately but were mild and irregular. Synto infusion was increased and when she was on the full whack (even after an hour) her contractions still were irregular and mild. So the decision was made to do a VE to check her progress. I did the VE and found she was 4-5cm dilated, partially effaced, the baby was OP (occipito posterior), with bulging membranes. Her waters had broken previously, but sometimes they can slide back in front of the baby's head. The midwife I was with advised me to break them, was what could be delaying the onset of good strong contractions, and I was just about to do that when they went spontaneously.

Was quite impressed with myself that I managed to feel the suture lines and fontanelle of the baby's head. Had not really felt these properly before and was able to feel them really well. So that was a first, and really boosted my confidence. As soon as the membranes had gone, things really started to hot up. Contractions immediately became stronger and more regular and she needed Entonox to cope with the pain. Two hours later she seemed to be involuntarily pushing at the peak of contractions and my mentor performed another VE to assess her progress. She was still 5-6cm dilated. This really knocked her down, and she became very tearful, but the contractions continued thick and fast and she was coping amazingly with it all; within half an hour she was pushing with all her might and the vertex (baby's head) was visible. As a para three (three previous babies) this was expected and I opened up my delivery pack and got my gloves on pretty sharpish! She pushed for about ten minutes, and then breathed a beautiful baby into the world. Baby delivered OP, so came out looking up at us all. I delivered her onto Mum's tummy, clamped the cord, gave Syntometrine to Mum, and Dad cut the cord.

Now, as soon as the baby's head was delivered I knew that something wasn't quite right. Baby looked distinctively like she had Down's Syndrome, but I didn't say anything straightaway. My mentor came back into the room and suggested I take the placenta to the sluice to check it, leaving Mum and Dad alone with their new baby for a few minutes. I loaded up my trolley and went to the sluice. My mentor asked if I was OK, and I just burst into tears . . . (felt so stupid), but I sobbed and sobbed and sobbed. In-between sobs I managed to get out that I thought the baby had Down's and mentor agreed. She gave me a big hug and said that we both needed to be strong for the parents, which I knew, but it was going to be hard.

I checked the placenta, and all was OK. Then we both went and spoke with the midwife in charge to let her know what was happening. She advised us to be open and honest with the parents and tell them that we suspected that the baby had Down's, and to offer them the opportunity to speak to a consultant paediatrician if they wanted to, but to do all the normal stuff like weighing the baby and offering vitamin K and completing initial baby check, like we would do anyway.

So I went off and got the weighing scales. Before we went back into the room my mentor squeezed my hand. Mum was holding the baby, and Dad was sitting next to her. My mentor initiated the conversation and said in a straightforward, open honest way that we thought the baby may have Down's, had they noticed this could be a possibility? They both said they had thought this. We offered the option of seeing the consultant paed, which they agreed to, and then I did all the normal baby bits.

The consultant paed came and spoke with them and after examining the baby, she agreed with the possible diagnosis of Down's. She explained that for it to be confirmed bloods would need to be sent, and that could be done in the morning. I helped Mum attach baby to the breast and she fed beautifully. The MCA had got them both tea and toast and we left them in peace to go and do all the paperwork. After a while I helped Mum into the shower and then we transferred her across to the ward. She had a side-room and Dad was allowed to stay overnight with her. As I was saying my goodbyes she gave me a huge hug and said she couldn't have got through it without me, and how special it was for me to be there with her. I felt so honoured, and just wanted to cry (again). I got home around 3a.m. and slept badly.

Got up this morning at 7.30a.m. to get the kids ready for school. There is a school service in the village church at 9.30a.m. I had promised to go because my daughter was reading a prayer at the end of the service. So walked them to school, they went on their bikes, and then nipped home for a quick cuppa before heading to the very cold village church. Thankfully the service only lasted thirty minutes; my hands hadn't quite turned to ice, but very nearly.

Still feel quite tearful and emotional now. After the wonderful feeling of being a midwife, knowing what to do, and being able to independently care for a woman in labour, the happiness, pride, worthiness, to the shock, sadness, disbelief, to the guilt for not being at home with my own children. Rang fellow student midwife, she was in the middle of a booking (oops), rang another fellow student midwife, and chatted to her for half an hour about it all. Felt good to talk about it. Need to distance myself somehow from those feelings and get back to my reality. Gym clothes were delivered this morning, don't feel like trying it all on but am going to make myself . . .

Friday

Didn't manage to try on my gym stuff yesterday. Had just gone upstairs when my mobile rang. It was delivery suite; one of my ladies was labouring! Midwife asked whether I wanted to go straight in or whether I wanted her to do VE and then let me know how she was progressing. Opted for her to do the VE, and ran upstairs to have a quick shower and wash my hair. Just got out the shower and the phone rang again, midwife had done VE and my lady was 5cm dilated and in the pool. Panic!!! Was 11.30a.m. Would she deliver before kids finished school? Would I be back in time to get them? Rang my brother and asked him to get kids from school if I wasn't home in time . . . And off I trotted back to the hospital, again (feel like I live there at the moment!).

Got to delivery suite, changed into scrubs, hair still dripping wet, but just tied it up in a ponytail, hadn't had a chance to straighten my fringe, and it was getting curlier and frizzier by the minute. My lady was still in the pool, and she was so pleased to see me when I went in (bless her). She introduced me to her hubby and then we sat and chatted. She was using hypno-birthing techniques for pain relief, and would stop when she got a contraction and shut her eyes, breathing it through. Then as soon as it had passed, she was happily chatting away again. Almost as soon as I went in she said she had a slight urge to push – talk about a good way to frighten a student midwife – ran and got midwife I was working with, and she calmly came and spent some time in the room with me!

After about an hour and a half my lady decided to get out of the pool, and use the active birthing bed, basically a double mattress on a low wooden platform. Had just taken some obs, and listened into the baby when her waters went. She started pushing. Within minutes her beautiful baby girl was born, and I lifted her up and put her onto Mummy's tummy for a cuddle. Cord was clamped, and Dad cut it, I sat and waited for the placenta to separate. Within a few minutes the placenta was delivered and I quickly examined her perineum; she had a couple of small labial grazes, but that was all. It was a beautiful, calm, serene delivery, and I felt really honoured to have been there with her. I told her that and we both had a few tears and a hug!

Completed all the paperwork, checked placenta. Was now 4p.m. and I was ready to go home. The midwife I was working with had been allocated the care of another lady who had just arrived. A first time mum who was in established labour and requiring pain relief. She did a VE and this lady was fully dilated! But, she wasn't having the urge to push, and the baby palpated OP . . . Knew this was going to be a long slog, and had to tell midwife that I couldn't stay, I needed to get back to my kids and hubby was working late, it wasn't fair for them to be at my brother's until the early hours of the morning (although I am sure they would have loved that!).

Midwife I was working with was great and sent me off to get my portfolio for her to sign. When I went down to the midwife station the other midwives were sitting there, and I told them that I was going. They all seemed rather indignant that I was passing on the opportunity to get another catch, saying (within my earshot) that if she doesn't want it, she doesn't want it and never known a student to pass on a catch before . . . wanted to shout at them all to make them understand. I had done a clinic the day before for five hours, had come back in and done nine and a half hours through the night, had four hours sleep and then been called back for another delivery, ending up on delivery suite for another six and a half hours . . . I was knackered, emotional from the Down's delivery, feeling under pressure to get my kids, and just needing to sit down and have a drink and eat something (seeing as the last time I had eaten or drunk anything was ten hours earlier at breakfast that morning). I tried explaining about the hours I had worked, and hubby working late and needing to get my children, but they didn't listen . . . Fuck 'em. Didn't care by this point. Said goodbye to my caseload lady and went to get my kids, got home an hour later and we all piled into bed (me with some cereal and a cuppa) and we chatted about their day at school, had a cuddle and watched some TV. Bliss!

Saturday

Turned my mobile off last night. Couldn't have coped with being called back in. Can't carry on like this . . . need some normality in my life. Midwife called within minutes of my phone being switched back on this morning. Did I want to meet her at one of my caseload ladies' house to remove the stitches from her emergency section wound. Knew I needed to get some postnatal visits for her in my portfolio so reluctantly agreed. Half-heartedly drove to her house and met midwife there, removed stitches; felt on auto-pilot . . . Only took fifteen minutes. When I left there I popped to hospital before coming home to see lady with Down's baby. She was doing well, although has had to cope with so much. Had a cuddle with her beautiful daughter whilst she told me that her hearing screen had been done and they thought she was deaf in one ear, her heart had been checked and she needed surgery (within a week) for a septal defect . . . just seemed like she had so much to deal with. Spent about an hour chatting to her, and they have adjusted to the situation brilliantly. Am sure if I were her, I wouldn't have coped as well as that.

Stopped at shop on way home and bought some nice bread rolls and a packet of bacon. Yummy! Also got some chocolate, needed to increase my blood sugar, seeing as I haven't eaten properly for a couple of days! Daughter is at a party this afternoon and I am taking son to local wildlife centre whilst she's out. Meant to be visiting family in London tomorrow, but they have forecast lots of snow, so will have to see . . .

Week Forty

Wednesday

Actually chanced taking my kids to visit family in London on Easter Sunday. Spent the whole day worrying whether my phone was going to ring. Have decided I hate being on-call, it mucks up my life! Can't do anything or go anywhere without feeling the fear of God that I will get called, and then have to drop everything and go to the hospital. Took my daughter to Mum's on Monday, again hoping and praying that my phone wouldn't go. Tuesday I took my little boy to the local wildlife centre, and we had been there about an hour when . . . yes, you know what happened! My phone rang. It was the husband of one of my ladies; they were on their way to the hospital. Now, had this been any lady I would have waited for labour to be confirmed by one of the midwives on delivery suite. However, this lady was a midwife, and therefore bloody well knew that she was in labour . . . just to add to the panic of needing to get to the hospital quickly, she had a history of very quick labours with her other kids (like thirty minutes) . . . So grabbed little boy who was staring at the tigers, ran back to car, frantically called my brother (who was on standby should this happen) and drove flat out, met my brother and little boy hopped into their car and went to spend the afternoon with them, and off I went to the hospital.

Walked onto delivery suite and one of the more senior midwives greeted me (warmly!) and told me to chuck my cardi and bags in the staff room and head straight for room ten. Was it that imminent? Burst into the room and my lady was on the CTG (previous section so high risk) and having a cannula sited because she had a low Hb. Very senior midwife was in there doing this, and she calmly said that I had time to go and get changed . . . so into scrubs I got, feeling the part now!

Back in the room, very senior midwife (who I have always been very frightened of) said she was going to go and sit outside and write up the notes, and that I should carry on. OK, can do this . . . monitored CTG, all looking good, lady not wanting any pain relief, just breathing through contractions. After twenty minutes or so I went and got very senior midwife, because I thought I could see some late decelerations on CTG. Late decelerations are a drop in the baby's heartrate to below 110bpm after the peak of a contraction, and can be a sign that the baby is starting to get distressed. She came and had a look and said that if they continued, we should offer to break her waters to speed things up a bit . . . She went off to handover and I carried on. Decelerations on CTG again, I knew she was handing over, so stuck my head out of the door and was lucky another senior midwife was just passing by so asked her to have a quick look. She couldn't work out whether they were decelerations or just good variability, and while we were looking the very senior midwife came back in. She couldn't decide either so the doctor was called to review (fat chance I have of ever interpreting a CTG if they can't!). Doctor said to ARM and continue to monitor, so very senior midwife ARM'd and I did a VE after. Lady was 5cm dilated. Very senior midwife announced she was going to have her lunch and told me to buzz her if I needed anything, and off she went. I can do this, I can do this, I can do this! My lady hit transition and was very seriously telling me that she had changed her mind, didn't want to go through labour anymore and was going home! Bless her . . . classic transition, even I recognised it. Then with the next contraction she got a bit pushy at the peak, held off on calling the very senior midwife away from her lunch, next contraction and a little more pushy . . . and again, so I pressed the buzzer. MCA came in and I asked her to get the very senior midwife for me because my lady was in the second stage. The very senior midwife returned (with a mouthful of something), looked at me, looked at lady and got her gloves on! I had prepared Syntometrine, and opened the delivery set and now put my gloves on too. Next push and the vertex was visible, and within what felt like seconds, but was actually about five minutes the baby's head was delivered. Could see cord wrapped tightly round baby's neck, and was able to get my finger underneath it and loosen it. Lovely restitution of baby's head, and then body was delivered, up onto Mum's tummy. Perfect!

The very senior midwife popped Syntometrine in for active third stage, I clamped cord and Dad cut cord . . . the placenta delivered, without any complications thankfully. Did all the paperwork, computer stuff and sorted out the six-hour discharge myself. Took a few hours, but the very senior midwife had finished her shift and had now gone, and everyone else was busy, so had to get on with it. Obviously did check everything I did with midwife in charge on the late shift.

The midwife I delivered the Down's baby with was on the late. She called me over at one point (in front of everyone) and asked me who my university tutor was. I told her. She asked me where my tutor was based, and I told her . . . (worried now!) and jokingly asked if she was going to write and complain about me! She said she felt I had handled the Down's situation so well that she wanted to write to my tutor and tell her what a wonderful midwife I am going to be, and what an asset to the team I will make. Nearly burst into tears again! Told her off for nearly making me cry in front of everyone, but thanked her.

Was home by 6p.m. Hubby had picked up little boy, and they had eaten fish and chips on the way home. Typical. I guess it would have been too much to ask for him to actually cook dinner himself. Daughter had phoned, so rang her at Mum's. She wanted me to take over some bits when I collect her. Told her that my lady had delivered and that her brother and I could spend Wednesday with them – she was not best impressed! She wanted to stay there on her own!

Well, have two more ladies due over the next week . . . only need one more caseload, but obviously every delivery counts (do need forty to qualify after all!). The advice I would give to all future student midwives is think things through more than I have. All my caseload ladies have been due over either the Christmas or Easter holidays. What should have been a lovely relaxing two-week holiday has not been that at all. I have been constantly looking at my mobile wondering when the next call will come. Moral of the story; make sure your caseload ladies are all due when you have your SCBU placement!

Friday

Not done anything midwifery for three days, must be a record! It's going to change now though. Have to crack on with the other essays I have to write. It's a miserable rainy day and kids are playing quite happily together (bloody miracle), so am going to write an essay plan for my neonatal essay. Have written the introduction already, and collected all the articles and policies I will use to reference my work. Just got to put it all together.

Had emailed my research essay to fellow student midwife who has a background of being a research nurse. She offered to read it for me, and emailed me back saying she was very impressed with it! Hope she really means it; did say that if it were utter rubbish I would prefer that she told me rather than lie.

Fellow midwife who failed the exam is coming over for dinner tonight with her hubby. After eating we are going to sit and do some revision together – her re-sit is only a week away.

Sunday

Clocks went forward this morning. Still wanted to be asleep, but was wide awake. Thought I would be aching all over after my induction at the gym yesterday. Yes, I finally made it there! A lovely lady showed me round; she did my blood pressure (105/58, not bad) and my weight 72kg (11st 3lb: very bad!). I did an hour on all sorts of gym equipment, and booked my next session for today. Took kids with me this morning, they can swim for free on my membership whilst I go to the gym. So had a thirty-minute session, just learning how to use more of the equipment. It was all the weight-type machines, and I can feel already that my arms and thighs are a bit wobbly from the work-out, am really going to suffer tomorrow.

Week Forty-one

Monday

Saw my caseload lady (the midwife) yesterday. Ended up chatting for an hour, and had a lovely cuddle with her baby son . . . even made me

feel a little broody (God, did I really just say that?!). Got home by
3.15p.m. and popped Sunday dinner in the oven. Kids were out on
the green playing with their friends and the phone rang. Hubby
answered and quickly handed it to me, it was delivery suite. One of
my caseload ladies was there, fully dilated, but not pushing, how fast
could I be there? Told her five minutes, grabbed bag and drove like a
maniac to the hospital.

Got there and found delivery suite heaving, midwife who was
handing over my lady was ending her shift and I took over with the
midwife in charge of shift supervising me. She also had a lady to care
for and was popping backwards and forwards to my lady's room,
checking we were OK. The plan was to start pushing as midwife who
had just left had done a VE and said she was fully dilated. So I talked
her through what to do and she started pushing. After twenty minutes
there was no sign of the baby's head, but I noticed a little trickle of
blood from her vagina. Called senior midwife immediately and informed
her. She stayed with me whilst I listened in to the baby's heart rate
(was doing this after every contraction anyway), as we were listening,
the baby's heart rate dropped significantly, but picked up again almost
straightaway. This was followed by a large blood clot being passed
from lady's vagina. Senior midwife immediately called for the doctors,
whilst I popped her onto a CTG so we could record the fetal heart
rate.

Further deep decelerations (of baby's heart) were heard along with
a further significant vaginal blood loss with numerous clots, and the
decision was made to perform an emergency Caesarean section. What
followed was a mad five minutes, in which time I had reassured her
that she was going to be OK whilst taking out her earrings, removing
her t-shirt and bra and popping a theatre gown on her. Another
wristband was written and put on, and the obstetric SHO (senior
house officer) sited a cannula . . . The SpR (specialist registrar) was
gaining consent for the EM LSCS (emergency lower segment Caesarean
section) and the anaesthetist was gaining consent for an epidural . . .
It was chaos! Bed was unplugged and we started for theatre at a run.
Senior midwife shouted that we needed CTG too, so I yelled at

anaesthetist to bring it with us. He looked a bit put out and said that he had stuff to prepare in theatre, but we were all going in the same bloody direction, and he did push it there for me. Senior midwife was in hysterics over what I had done; she meant to ask my lady's partner to push it for us, not the consultant anaesthetist! Who cares, just because he is a consultant doesn't mean he can't help with things like that . . . People treat them like God, and then they get this all high and mighty attitude – not me, treat them the same as everyone else, I do! So, now we are in theatre. Epidural is sited quickly. Urinary catheter is inserted. Fetal heart keeps dropping. I am scrubbed ready to take the baby. The senior midwife leaves theatre to bleep the paeds. The baby is delivered and handed to me . . . baby is flat and floppy . . . no signs of life, dreadful colour (white), no respiratory effort, covered in meconium and blood . . . FUCK . . . Shout at runner in theatre to get midwife. Put the baby on Resuscitaire, suction meconium from mouth, rub dry to try and stimulate breathing. Midwife back, takes over . . . still no paed . . . I am sent to find paed. Yell at MCA to bleep paed again, check in changing room, check in SCBU, back in corridor outside theatre and paed saunters through from main theatres . . . I yell at her to get into theatre and she runs in to take over. Baby had pinked up and was now crying . . . Thank God. Never, ever want to repeat that, thank you very much. She had a major placental abruption, which is when the placenta separates from the uterus before the baby is delivered. It can be life-threatening for the mum and the baby . . . Was horrendous. Provided all the post-op care (can do that bit, was my job after all). Senior midwife was handing over and I sat and chatted to MCA. When she'd finished handing over she came over and asked me if I was due to qualify in the summer, and when I told her I don't qualify for another nine months she was surprised! She asked if I wanted to work there, and I told her I was hoping I would be offered a job . . . She said that she thought they would offer me a job as she thought I fitted in very well, and she hadn't heard anyone saying anything nasty about me! Now, I know I am insecure, so hearing this just made me feel so much better, especially as she's the delivery suite manager!

Wrote it all up in my portfolio and got senior midwife to sign everything. We sat down and had a cuppa and talked over what had just happened. Lady had a placental abruption, was losing blood, and the baby was therefore suffering. She praised me for how calm I had stayed, and said that I had done all the right things; made me feel better because at the time I had wanted to cry! Got home around 9p.m. Kids asleep in bed. Hubby in a strop because I had been called out again. The joys of being a student midwife.

Spent today back at uni. Strange being in a classroom again, seems like ages since I have done that. Was very boring. We were given yet another presentation to prepare so had better crack on and get it done. That way I can have tomorrow to play with the kids all day!

Tuesday

The kids have been driving me up the wall today, bless them. They have been arguing and just being silly. So, after feeding them up with a big lunch I decided to take them and the dog for a walk in the park.

No sooner had we got there than my mobile rang. Delivery suite. One of my ladies had just arrived . . . could I make my way there? Told the midwife I would need to sort out childcare because the children were still on their Easter holidays, and that I would phone back and let them know what was happening. Awful really, because I didn't have any intention of going in. Sounds cruel, but this particular lady I had only met once, and I have sacrificed enough of my family life recently. So, carried on walking around the park with kids and dog, and after half an hour rang back and made my apologies to delivery suite. They said I should ring when hubby got home from work to see if she was still labouring and go in then if she was. Afternoon was spoilt by it; felt guilty, felt awful for not being there, felt worried what all the midwives would think.

Hubby got home around 4p.m. and I dutifully rang delivery suite. My lady had delivered soon after arriving, so there was no panic to suddenly get there quickly. Sorted hubby and kids with some dinner and then made my way to my hypno-birthing lady for a postnatal visit (officially a social visit because I was going alone, without my mentor). Got there around 5.30p.m. and sat and chatted for what felt like hours (was about an hour in the end). Had a lovely cuddle with her beautiful baby girl, and my lady quite happily reflected on her birth experience with me. She was very positive about the whole thing, which was fabulous! She gave me a lovely handmade card, with my photograph on the front, holding her baby, and a lovely message inside asking me to be there for baby number three! Also got some yummy chocolates (well, do go to the gym now after all, so the odd box of chocolates will be OK! Hee hee hee . . .)

Wednesday

Was a long day at uni, presentation went OK, but quite emotional too. Our cohort leader retired today. She has always been the one who has looked out for our group; we are the last lot in the uni doing the eighteen-month midwifery conversion programme, all the others are three-year direct entry girls, and the other lecturers seem to favour them . . . meaning we are left to muddle through best we can . . . never mind. So, she left, not there anymore; had a laugh through the day, and got to know a bit more of the real her! We will all miss her greatly. Very sad.

My mobile rang later that evening. It was my community mentor, asking if I was OK! Odd . . . Had a chat, and she said she was impressed by all my ladies' comments about me. That they had all been saying very complimentary things (Good, good! Sigh of relief!!) She mentioned she had been and done a home visit on my placental abruption flat baby caseload lady, and explained that this lady was very unhappy with her experience, because she didn't understand what had happened to her, and that she had felt the postnatal care in the hospital had been poor. I was horrified. I felt I had talked her and her husband through everything as it was happening, in an attempt to prevent them from feeling like this afterwards. Anyway, I explained to my mentor what had happened, and said that I was going to see her anyway for a postnatal visit, and I would make sure I gave her the opportunity to ask questions. That way I could try and explain what had happened and why. Rang her as soon as I had finished speaking to mentor, and arranged to see her tomorrow at 5p.m.

Thursday

Woke up to find one of my caseload ladies had sent me a text me last night. She said to look out for her baby's birth announcement in the local newspaper. The paper was popped through the door this afternoon, and I looked through it trying to find the page with the birth announcements on it . . . there is was. Her and her partner's names, baby's name, date of birth, time of birth, weight . . . and there was my name! It said special thanks to midwife ME! Am so proud. Text her to say thank you, then text every single person on my phone telling them to look in local paper at birth announcements! Have cut it out, and popped it in envelope with the card and photos she gave me. Am going to buy a little box to keep these keepsakes in. What a lovely thought on her part!

Placental abruption flat baby caseload lady rang at 4p.m. and cancelled my visit for this evening. Am going tomorrow instead.

Friday

New carpet being laid today. Took forever to move all the stuff out of the living room last night. Finished the last bit off this morning. Just hope it doesn't rain, because the sofas are on the patio! It is an afternoon fitting so that means they could arrive anytime between 12p.m. and 5p.m. It's 1.30 already, so am hoping they get here quickly. Probably take me forever to get all the stuff back into the living room!

Really feel like I have had the chance to have a proper break now that my caseload ladies have all delivered. Am still doing the odd postnatal visit to ensure my portfolio is complete, but it's nothing like being on-call. Went to the gym again this morning and they have now put together a programme for me to complete every time I go. It will take an hour and fifteen minutes each time, and they want me to do it at least three times a week! Well, if I do it on a Saturday and a Sunday then I will only have to fit it in once during the week itself; that's the plan anyway! Kids went into the pool whilst I got that sorted, and I go back tomorrow to actually do this programme for the first time! Yikes!

Have been doing a bit of midwifery stuff too. Have now got my neonatal essay planned (have been doing that in bed the last couple of evenings, hubby isn't best impressed!). Am writing it on how to test that a NG tube is in the correct location before giving a feed through it. There is plenty of literature out there on this, and I have read through a lot of it, highlighting bits ready to use in the essay. Just have to sit down and write it now! Kids go back to school on Tuesday, so after I have been to the gym I will sit down and make a proper start on it. Still need to tweak the research one too. But plan to do that tonight so it's completely finished – about time too! Went to see placental abruption lady this evening. Was awful. She sat there and cried. She said every time she thinks back to her labour and birth she cries uncontrollably. She didn't understand what had happened to her, and why she had to have an emergency section. Tried to explain as best I could everything that had happened. They were very kind to me, saying there wasn't anything I could have done differently, and that they were happy with the care I had provided. But they were very angry with the midwife in charge who (quite rightly, which I tried my best to explain) refused entry to her family when she was in recovery. Spent a lot of time promoting the birth afterthoughts service at the hospital and was encouraged to hear that she was going to contact them to make an appointment. That way she could speak to an experienced midwife, have all her questions answered, and have counselling at the same time. Anyway, left after an hour, drove round the corner, and just sat and cried. Pulled myself together and went home (to my beautiful new carpet); back to mother/wife mode.

Week Forty-two

Monday

Re-sit day for fellow student midwife. Couldn't bear the thought of her being alone waiting to go into the exam. I set alarm for 6.30a.m. and dragged kids out of bed at 7a.m. We set off for uni at 7.45a.m. only to be sat in traffic for what seemed like forever, with two grumpy kids in the car. Oh joy!

We all got there in the end and I bought her a cuppa, and sat and tried to reassure her that she would be OK. Tutor was a bit off with us for being there to support her, but don't give a flying fuck what she thinks. Anyway, left fellow student midwife in tears, just about to start re-sit and tutor shut the classroom door. Had two and a half hours to kill; car needed two new tyres – that took an hour. Took kids to big activity centre to play – that was another hour. I sat and read through the other girls' research essays that they had sent me to comment on (why they sent it to me I will never know, did tell them I was crap at research but hey ho). Then headed back to uni to be there in time for the end of the exam. She came out looking quite confident that she had done well, and described the questions as being easy. Fingers crossed she gets through. By this time the kids were starving, so we popped to supermarket to get some lunch. Had promised them that we could go to the swimming pool for the inflatable fun session, so off we went. I went into the gym whilst they went into the pool. Third day in a row that I have managed to do my workout programme, can run for four minutes now without feeling like I am going to pass out! Was then a mad dash to get to the doctor's from there. Daughter has funny itchy spots on back of her knees, molluscum contagiosum apparently. You just have to wait for it to go away on its own . . . great! Finally got home at 3.30p.m. Feel knackered. Kids are back at school tomorrow (finally) after the very long Easter holidays, so will have to make myself get back into a routine with working through the day when I have private study days. Have three essays due in, and only seven weeks to do them all. Usually takes me a month to do one! Shit!

Tuesday

Have had a busy day, again. Don't seem to get to relax properly these days. Dropped kids off at school and went straight to the gym. Finished my workout by 10.45a.m. and after a quick shower, drove to see my lady who had had the Down's baby. Was so nice to see her, and sit and have a chat. She reflected on her birthing experience with me and described my care as wonderful and that even my voice was calming! Really needed that boost (after my placental abruption lady had sat and sobbed when reflecting on her birth experience last week, been feeling rubbish ever since). She also gave me the most beautiful hand-made card with a photo of me holding her gorgeous daughter on the front, which her older daughter had made for me. Said my goodbyes and got in the car ready to head home. Got a text message from my community mentor. It said 'The health visitor asked me to pass on to you all the great feedback that she has received from your ladies. They are all thrilled you were there and with your care. Keep up the good work. Well done!' Felt much better already! Drove home with a huge grin on my face.

Spent the afternoon editing my fellow student midwife's research essay. Took a long time, but we got there in the end. After a trip to the dentist with the kids I was back home reading another fellow student's research essay. Don't mind helping, but haven't had a chance to do anything to my own neonatal essay (which was the original plan for today).

Wednesday

Oh my God . . . don't know where to start. Had a full day in uni today, with the slightly ditsy lecturer, focusing on alternative therapies and massage. Started well; we all actually managed to control our giggles for the first hour and twenty minutes, only had ten minutes to go till coffee, but I just couldn't stop myself. Lecturer was talking about Bach Flower Remedies, and in a very matter-of-fact way said something along the lines of Bach Flower Remedies were established by – 'umm, rrrrrrrrr, umm' – Bach! It was so funny, just the way she said it and the matter of fact tones she used. Burst out laughing, the others were all sniggering behind hands . . . tried to turn the laugh into a cough and failed miserably, so just ran from the room making really odd noises . . . lecturer thought I was choking . . . other girls by this point were on the floor wetting themselves with laughter. Had tears streaming down my face by now, and got some really odd looks from some of the other students on campus. Made it to the toilet and had to splash cold water on my face to calm down. Returned to the room a few minutes later with a glass of water. Didn't dare make eye contact with anyone.

The rest of the day wasn't much better; we all had intermittent giggling episodes, which the lecturer either failed to notice or chose to ignore. We learnt how to massage each other's hands, then I volunteered to have my feet massaged . . . was lovely, so relaxing. Then we were given life-sized dolls to practise neonatal massage on. That was it; we were all off again. Trying to see through the tears, I was sitting on the floor with a baby (doll) in front of me, asking it whether it was OK to perform a massage; the lecturer told us that gaining consent is very important in healthcare, that even newborns can communicate whether they are happy for you to massage them. OK, have now died, and ended up in some obscure alternative dimension. Managed (somehow) to perform a thirty-minute massage on a plastic doll. Is this what I signed up for?

Got home and rang delivery suite to sort out my off-duty. Have another two-week placement there starting soon. Can't wait – love it so much! Have just been emailed another fellow student's research essay; she wants 700 words removed as it's over the limit, so am going to try and do that now. Really want to get to the gym this evening, but peak time is up till about 8p.m. and don't want to go when it's busy, but after that is too late. Not going to go after dropping the kids off at school in the morning because it's also too busy that time of day. Will aim for lunchtime tomorrow; the bloke in the gym said it was quieter then, so will give it a go. Feel guilty at not going today though. Shouldn't, because they said to aim to do the workout three times a week and I have now done it four days in a row . . . hopefully I will have started to lose some weight soon. Can't believe I weighed over eleven stone. Yikes! Really need to crack on with this neonatal essay, seeing as I got the whole library's supply of neonatal textbooks out today!

Week Forty-three

Monday

Have had yet another roller-coaster week . . . seriously think they should put a health warning on this midwifery degree lark. After a couple of incidences with my little boy at school last week, I had decided to quit the course and be a stay-at-home mum. Got the guilt complex, that I need to be at home to be a good mum. Utter rubbish obviously! Anyway, still struggling with my feelings as far as that is concerned. Had got it all planned (again), how I would manage with no income, possibly going back to theatres for one day per week, concentrating on being a mother. Son has mild ADHD, which at least has been diagnosed now. School haven't done a thing to acknowledge this, and are still treating him as the naughty boy . . . doesn't help. Daughter is probably feeling completely ignored, bless her, and as for hubby – can't bear the sight of him.

Feel like I have so much to do, and no time or space to do it. Research essay was handed it at uni this morning (finally), but then I had to come home, missing the afternoon lectures. Sister-in-law's car broke down last week, so she cannot collect kids from school for me.

Brother is in Sri Lanka; she has no way of getting out and about. I have no childcare. Have missed lecture outlining the next essay. It's raining buckets. Have just paid £150 (which I haven't got) for sister-in-law to have a hire car for a week. Was on phone to hire car people for ages and now don't have enough time to go to the gym. Have three essays to write in six weeks whilst going to uni and working full-time, and now it's hailing . . . Urrrggghhh! Maybe this is why there aren't enough midwives; sane people quit before they qualify.

Wednesday

Yesterday was a day well spent! Got up and remembered a dream which completely planned my complex midwifery care analysis! How utterly fabulous is that? Grabbed some paper and wrote my essay plan in thirty seconds flat. Even have most of the research I will need already. Result! Took kids to school, met sister-in-law at car hire place and sorted car for her (very jealous – it's brand new, she is the first person to drive it and it's gorgeous!); went to gym; came home; wrote my neonatal essay; collected kids from school; got called into school (again). Got into classroom and son's teacher (supply teacher he has once a week, and generally comes home moaning about) was waiting for me. OK, deep breath, let's hear it – what an awful mother I must be to have such an unruly child. What I actually heard next knocked me for six. What a wonderfully well-behaved son I have, and how he worked so hard this afternoon in music. Eyes welled up with tears, and could have hugged the teacher. What a pleasant change to hear something positive!

Once kids were in bed (and they both went to sleep straightaway; I must have entered the Twilight Zone yesterday, I tell you) I carried on with my essay, with aching knees (don't know what I did wrong at the gym, but my legs hurt).

Today was quite a draining day at uni. Spent all day learning about the hypertensive disorders of pregnancy (pre-eclampsia, eclampsia . . . and HELLP syndrome), felt like shouting HELP at the top of my voice by the end of it. Legs still hurt too, to the point I have been taking ibuprofen all day, and am not going to the gym tonight. Got home to find the house empty. Panicked, thinking sister-in-law had forgotten to get the kids from school. She had actually forgotten the door key, and had driven all the way home (twenty minutes) and back again (another twenty minutes) to get the key, not realising that my father-in-law, next door but one, has a spare key. She knows now. Made use of the peace and quiet and rang delivery suite; have sorted my off-duty for my two weeks on there, so can plan my childcare now. Son arrived home first; he had another good day at school, even getting a merit! Daughter was off running a cross-country race for the school. Hubby not back from working away, yippee!

By 7p.m. the house was full. Everyone home. Everyone fed. Everyone bathed. By 8p.m. kids in bed. By 9p.m. unfortunately hubby home too. I have managed to write more of my neonatal essay. Just got to tidy it up a bit and it's done. Will aim to do that tomorrow night. Now 10p.m. and bedtime for me too.

Thursday

Had a whole day of airy-fairy lecturer today. We were all dreading it, and were all desperate not to be reduced to fits of hysterical laughter. Rather surprisingly, I found the day was actually very beneficial. We recapped on our knowledge as nurses discussing venepuncture and cannulation. Then practiced for a bit on rubber arms. I do it quite a lot now when I am on placement – venepuncture that is, but was fun stabbing rubber arms and squirting fake blood everywhere!

One of the girls couldn't get the fake blood out of her rubber arm, so I offered my own arm. Have huge juicy veins, so they are really good to practise on. She missed, bless her.

I practised siting a cannula. Have only attempted that once in practice so far and failed. So actually, did need the practice. Got one in the rubber arm first attempt, was well pleased. Fake blood pouring all over the place, but cannula was in! Airy-fairy lecturer waited until fake blood was all over our hands, clothes, table and floor before deciding to tell us it stains. So have pink splodges on my skin . . . fetching – not!

The afternoon was taken up with the topic of water birth. We discussed it to death, although did watch an amazing video, and looked at some beautiful photographs of babies emerging through the water into the world. Hope I get to deliver a water birth soon, think it would be a fantastic experience. So, had got to the middle of the afternoon, no-one had had any hysterical bursts of laughter, and airy-fairy lecturer had not said anything dumb to trigger us off, apart from continually saying 'Am I OK?', to which I just wanted to say 'Well actually no, you're not, you're completely off your fucking rocker', just to see her reaction. By this point I had tuned out from listening to her, and was deep in conversation with my fellow student midwife about her unfortunate morning . . . she had put diesel in her petrol car, which had subsequently started smoking like a chimney and conked out in the middle of a very busy roundabout, halting rush-hour traffic, until a lorry driver pushed her car onto the grassy roundabout, at which point she stood there watching the rush hour traffic go by, wondering what the hell she was going to do. To cut a long story short, her £30 tank of diesel ended up costing another £150 to get it all drained out and the engine working again . . . ouch! Whilst we were chatting I rocked back on my chair, and nearly fell off backwards; that got the others laughing hysterically, then I realised I had a label hanging out of the back of my trousers, which after further investigation turned out to be coming out of my knickers which were on inside-out. Like to share these things with the group, so announced this to them, hysterical laughter (again) followed. I had answered the lecturer's water birth question with the answer my knickers are on inside-out . . . oops!

Got home to two beautifully behaved angels (someone else's kids in disguise, obviously). At this moment they are snuggled up on the sofa watching a DVD with hubby. I am supposed to be finishing off my essay, just preparing myself for the final onslaught. Knees still no better by the way. Might ring gym tomorrow and ask their advice if they still hurt. Can't keep taking ibuprofen, and I want to keep up with my three times a week pact I made with myself. Only been once so far this week, and it's Thursday already . . . doesn't bode well really does it?

Friday

Whole day of blood, with lecturer who is very A&P orientated. Two fellow midwives pulled a bunk and didn't even bother coming. Started with revision of blood and its constituents, and then moved on to anaemia and understanding blood results. Was boring . . . lecturer hadn't done any prep (and it was blatantly obvious). Was a shambles actually. Could have used the time better at home working on my essay. Only saving grace of the day was getting to the library at lunchtime and getting out all the books I need for my complex midwifery care analysis. Don't think I will be doing it on anaemia after today's lecture though, all a bit too complex for my liking. Lecturer gave it up as a bad job by 2.30p.m. and we escaped.

Fantastic, we were on our way home, looking forward to a long weekend and then delivery suite next week. Stopped off at supermarket as fellow student midwife who was driving needed to get a cheap top for her evening out tonight. Tried loads on, she got a gorgeous one, but I was very self-controlled and didn't spend a penny. Back in car on way home by 3.30p.m. Just about to overtake a car when this weird noise started, and a strong smell of burning rubber filled the car . . . engine promptly cut out and we coasted into a lay-by. Couldn't find hazard lights initially, but got them on, then looked under car to find out what was making that noise. Looked like lots of wires hanging down. Tried to open bonnet but didn't know how, and when we found the right lever it didn't work. PANIC! Fellow student midwife had breakdown cover but couldn't remember who it was with. By chance I still had my breakdown cover details in my uni bag after getting it out of my own car on Thursday after the diesel incident, and it happened to jog fellow student midwife's memory that she was with the same people and she rang them. Someone would be with us within thirty minutes . . . we waited . . . he arrived, was cam belt (?) that had broken and he couldn't fix it next to the roadside, he would have to arrange for a flatbed truck to come out and recover us. He drove off . . . we waited . . . and waited . . . and waited . . . an hour and a half later the flatbed truck arrived . . . the bloke agreed to drop me off at home en route to garage near fellow student midwife's home. Now 6.30p.m. and have just walked through the door.

Plan is to try (yet again) to finish neonatal essay. Am knackered though, so not holding out much hope that I will manage to do anything apart from veg on the sofa!

Saturday – otherwise known as knee crisis day

Got up early as having a TV unit delivered. You know what they are like; 'We will deliver anytime between 7.30a.m. and 1p.m.' – fantastic. Was lucky. They delivered at 9.30a.m. so managed to get to the supermarket this morning to do weekly food shop, horrendous on a Saturday morning at the best of times due to far too many people . . . trolley rage! Anyway, got halfway round and could barely walk, my knees were hurting so much. Had to abandon my shopping trolley and come home and ring the doctor. Because it's a Saturday, it was the emergency doctor I had to call, and got fobbed off by a patronising triage nurse who basically said they couldn't do anything, keep taking ibuprofen and stop going to the gym . . . thanks love, that was helpful (not). So have been dosed up to the eyeballs on ibuprofen. My little bro popped in and recommended glucosamine. I had never heard of it, but he takes it. Apparently we have a family history of incredibly bad joints – news to me!

Anyway, sad cow that I am, kids and hubby have gone off to a friend's fortieth birthday party (sixties-themed fancy dress) and I have stayed home to finish my neonatal essay, which . . . fanfare please . . . I have just finished! Hooray!!! No more having to think back to that bloody long six-week SCBU placement . . . I am freeeee!

It's just gone 9p.m., they are still at the party, and I am going to open my bottle of red wine and enjoy having the TV remote all to myself on a Saturday night. What a treat. Can have a day off tomorrow, and then start on the complex midwifery care analysis on Monday. Sorted.

Week Forty-three

Monday

Rubbish start to the week. Took kids to school and was informed by before and after school club that son had been in a fight last Friday morning after I dropped them off. What am I supposed to do to bring his behaviour into line? Have phoned the school nurse and asked for one-to-one behavioural support sessions, which she had offered to do when I saw her a few months ago. Just waiting for her to call me back. Amazing how I can go from feeling so positive to feeling so down and depressed so quickly.

Tuesday

Got lots done on my essay yesterday. Also saw doctor about knees, he said it was a gym injury (no shit Sherlock), and referred me to a physio, who can't see me for a week (bloody NHS). Did get some mega-strong painkillers.

So, was back on delivery suite from this morning. Got up at 6a.m. ready to be at work for 7.30. Got to work and listened to handover, and all ladies on delivery suite were not doing a lot . . . were in latent labour, or had come in for assessments and were being sent home. So much for me getting more deliveries. The midwife in charge asked me what I wanted from my placement, and I said deliveries, to which the midwife in charge of the night shift laughed and said there was no chance. Not to be deterred, I took over the care of a lady who had come in at 6a.m. claiming to be in labour. She apparently put on her self-hypnosis tape and immediately went into a hypnotic state, which she was still in! When we entered the room, this horrendously awful spa treatment-type music was playing in the background. I stood and watched her for a while, then feeling almost like I was intruding I asked if I could feel her tummy to gain an idea of the regularity and strength of her contractions. They were whopping great huge ones, lasting about ninety seconds, very strong to palpate, and coming regularly every three minutes. I took a set of observations. My mentor said we should do a VE to see what she was up to, and if she was in labour at all, because if she wasn't she needed to go home! So I did a VE. Now, I am not the expert when it comes to these things, and I felt the cervix, and just double-checked it too . . . she was 8cms dilated! Couldn't believe it! She remained in this trance-like state for about an hour. I popped out of the room for a cuppa, returning ten minutes later to find her on all fours swaying and really breathing through the contractions. I asked her if she wanted Entonox and she agreed. My mentor popped in and said she was transferring a lady to the ward, and if I needed anything just to press the buzzer . . . OK, time for student midwife to panic . . . no sooner had mentor gone when lady started to push involuntarily with her contractions. When the contraction finished, I asked her if she was aware of the urge to push and she said she was, so I encouraged her to listen to her body and to start pushing if that's what she wanted to do. Next contraction came and boy did she start pushing! There's me, hurtling round the room trying to get everything ready – delivery set, Syntometrine, Resuscitaire, towels – and she is quite happily pushing away! Pressed the buzzer to get a midwife in the room with me. MCA came, and I asked her to get me a midwife. Midwife in charge came in because my mentor was still on the ward. Felt a bit under pressure then (no reason to because she is lovely and very much a normality midwife). My mentor returned after a couple of minutes, just in time. Vertex was now visible at the peak of pushes, and within ten minutes of the onset of the second stage, I caught a gorgeous little boy . . . it was perfect! Catch number sixteen!

It's so special to see a new family together for the first time. We left them to it to head to the sluice and check the placenta. Midwife I was working with got called into another room, and I completed all the paperwork, put all the details on the computer, weighed the baby, gave vitamin K etc. and transferred her to the ward. It was now lunchtime and the afternoon girls had come on, so I sat and had lunch. Not much to do. Helped transfer a couple of ladies across to the ward. Then midwife I had been working with said we were being allocated to a lady who had Prostin at midday and was ARM-able (her waters could be broken to help kick-start labour). She was twelve days overdue so was being induced. So at 3p.m. I went and got her from the ward. She was having good strong regular contractions, and coping well using Entonox. At 3.15 I performed an ARM; she was 5cm dilated, and the baby was direct OP. It was 3.30 and my shift was ending, but I decided to stay on for a bit because things had really kicked off and the birth looked imminent. She was bouncing on her birthing ball, and not able to find a position that was comfortable at all. She was demanding pain relief, and was becoming increasingly aggressive. I tried to calm her down and reassure her, but the situation wasn't helped by an equally aggressive partner and mother-in-law also demanding pain relief for her. Then she started throwing herself around the bed, and I just knew she'd hit transition. I was right! Ten minutes later her bouncing baby boy came into the world! Seventeenth catch and second of the day! Wow . . . how wrong was last night's midwife in charge! Did feel slightly guilty; there was a three-year direct entry student midwife on the afternoon shift who only has two catches so far. Her lady had needed an instrumental this afternoon, and if I had gone home when my shift ended, she would have got my catch, but then again, she still has two and a half years of training left, and I only have eight months. She will easily get her catches in that time, whereas me getting another twenty-three in the six weeks I have left on delivery suite is going to be tight.

So, got home a little late, very tired and incredibly happy. Seventeen catches! Wow . . . am buzzing! Little boy has been good today (bloody miracle) and has been playing beautifully out the front with the neighbour's children all evening. It's the first summery evening of spring, and it's gorgeous outside. Might go and sit in the garden myself actually!

Wednesday

Forgot to turn my alarm off last night, so was rudely awoken at 6a.m. this morning. Did go back to sleep but now have huge bags under my eyes! Son was in an argumentative mood. He wanted to wear shorts because it had been so hot yesterday, but is quite chilly today, and rain is forecast, which I tried to explain, but he went off on one. Then when we got to school he refused to take his proper place in the line. Am now dreading him being there, I just know he is going to have a naughty day.

I should be writing my essay. Start work at 1.30p.m. so that gives me three hours to work on essay and one hour to get ready and get to work . . . that's the plan anyway.

10.30a.m.

Just been making a cuppa and reflecting on my fantastic day yesterday. All the midwives, when introducing me to the women, referred to me as one of our senior student midwives! How fabulous is that? Haven't quite got it into my head that I am a student midwife at all, but am already a senior student midwife! Have actually been working on my essay too . . . it's coming together slowly. I know what I want to write, it's just getting the words right to make it flow, and choosing which references to use; takes me forever to write an essay. But I normally get good grades, so I guess the effort is worthwhile.

Thursday

Looked after a wonderful couple on delivery suite yesterday. It was her second baby, although she had not laboured before because her first baby had been breech and she had an elective Caesarean. She was huffing and puffing away when I took over, using her Entonox and about to have an epidural sited. Once the epidural was in, she was immediately more comfortable, and I then spent the next eight hours chatting to her! Obviously I did some work too. Obs were recorded, she was on a CTG so I kept an eye on that, because of the epidural she had a catheter and I emptied that a couple of times. Did a couple of VEs; she was dilating very slowly and her pubic arch was very low, so there was a worry that the baby wouldn't be able to pass through her pelvis. Anyway, about an hour before the end of my shift the doctors came to review her, and by this point her contractions had started to become irregular. Doc did a VE and she was still 9cm dilated; doc got her to push with a contraction to see if anterior lip of cervix could be pushed over the baby's head but it couldn't, so the decision was made to perform an EM LSCS (emergency Caesarean section) for failure to progress. The selfish student midwife in me was gutted, I had provided all this care, and wasn't going to be able to put her in my portfolio because it was a section not a vaginal delivery . . . gutted. She was being wheeled into theatre just as my shift was ending, but her partner asked if I would stay with them, so I did. Dutifully I scrubbed and caught the baby, a little girl (we were all sure it was going to be a little boy!). She was beautiful, with huge eyes, very alert, looking round at us all! I stayed until she was transferred into recovery, and then made my way home. The house was in darkness, and everyone was asleep. Made myself a cuppa, and chilled out watching TV for half an hour before heading up to bed.

Did not want to get up this morning. Goodness knows how I will feel tomorrow morning, as I am doing a late today, and then an early tomorrow. Anyway, plan is to try and do some more of my essay, get a little bit done every day! Was hoping to have heard from fellow student midwife who failed her exam; she was told to expect her results two weeks after the re-sit and it was two weeks on Monday. She has sent me a text about work but not mentioned the exam results – keeping my fingers crossed for her.

10.30p.m.

Got to work and midwife in charge gave me the joint care of two ladies who she thought would deliver on my shift. Tried to spend equal time with both of them; each was about 5cm dilated. Only three midwives on delivery suite, due to sick leave. Within the space of an hour or so, the ward was full of labouring women. Community midwives were being called in, midwives were being pinched from the postnatal ward, big boss midwives were having to work hands-on. Then there was a shoulder dystocia in the pool . . . it was chaos.

Anyway, I did a VE on one of my ladies and she was still 9cm dilated, four hours after she was 8cm dilated . . . doctors got involved and it was decided they would do an EM LSCS (emergency Caesarean section) for failure to progress. So off to theatre we went. Caught her chubby little girl (best part of 10lb!) and had just transferred Mum back to recovery bay when my shift was over. Said my goodbyes to her, and to the other lady (who was still 8cm at that point) and came home, tired, very hungry, in need of a lot of sleep, and disappointed that neither of my ladies had delivered vaginally.

Friday

As predicted, I did not want to get out of bed this morning. When I managed to drag myself out, I made the mistake of looking in the mirror. To say my eyes were puffy is an understatement! Made it to work with ten minutes spare to get changed and bloody stupid car parking machine wouldn't accept my money. Makes me sooo mad that I have to pay to park at the hospital anyway, seeing as I work there, and it's too far to walk or cycle to, and the buses don't run through my village at the right times to get me to work. So, bloody machine kept giving me my money back. It's a £35 fine for not paying, so I found an old receipt in my car and scribbled a note on the back explaining that I had tried to get a ticket, but bloody machine wouldn't accept my money and I would ring the general office at 9a.m. to tell them.

Sat listening to handover. Only labouring woman was a twenty-seven weeker whose baby had passed away. It wasn't deemed appropriate for me to care for her as a student (although it will be expected of me as a qualified midwife), so I was given a lady who had come in with grade two meconium (mec) stained liquor with no contractions. She was a very precious young girl. Everything was too much or too painful for her. Siting an IV was like, well, I've never seen anyone make such a fuss before. Docs decided that due to mec (she was only 3cm dilated) she needed augmentation so IV Synto was started and an epidural was sited. She was labouring quite nicely when midwife in charge came to find me to say there was a para two (lady who'd had two babies previously) who had SROM'd (spontaneous rupture of membranes) on her way in and would I like to care for her . . . Course I would!

Lady arrived a while later, and midwife in charge was busy so I took her to her room and took a history and her observations. She was having moderate contractions every five minutes, which were lasting about thirty seconds. She was asking for pain relief and we tried some Entonox, but she didn't like the way it made her feel. Midwife in charge came in at this point, and instead of asking me what we had been discussing, or reading the notes I had written, proceeded to ask all the same questions again. I did butt in and say we had discussed this, but she ignored me and carried on (bitch). Then she proceeded to make me do another abdominal palpation in front of her, whilst she asked me the most awkward questions. I also had to use a pinard (never heard a heartbeat through one yet) before she repeated the palpation again. Thank the Lord I got it all right. I actually managed to hear a heartbeat using a pinard (there is a God). She then praised me for getting it all right, and suggested I make the couple some tea.

Outside the room she gave me a bollocking for offering Entonox without her permission, adding 'It is a drug you know!' I know! But she wasn't offering this poor woman any pain relief and she was obviously in a lot of discomfort, and trying to cope, perhaps if she had been screaming and been vocal it would have been different. Makes me know what sort of midwife I want to be when I qualify! So, was in and out of the room for an hour or so, contractions were hotting up. She then became more assertive and asked directly for pain relief. Midwife in charge was about to start handover (takes thirty minutes), she wasn't convinced that this lady was in labour and basically suggested I sit in room with lady, observing contractions and explain that a VE was necessary before stronger pain relief could be given; delay tactics, makes me mad. So off I trotted. By the time the afternoon midwife came on, lady was really working hard with her contractions. I handed over from my point of view and we did a VE together straightaway. She was 6cm dilated, and head was at the spines . . . not in labour huh? Screw you, senior midwife! We gave her a shot of Meptid and she chilled out for a while. Midwife went off to do computer bits and I stayed in the room keeping the partogram up to date, listening into the fetal heart and rubbing her back through the contractions. At 3p.m. she said she wanted to push, so I buzzed for the midwife. As the midwife came into the room I updated her and said I would get the delivery set open, but she said no. She didn't think the lady would deliver that quickly. Next contraction came, and she was definitely pushing, lots of anal dilatation and vertex was visible! Grabbed my gloves, opened my delivery set and crouched down on the floor ready to catch (she was standing on a mat leaning over the bed for support). Next contraction and the baby was delivered straight into my waiting hands! Lovely little girl . . . Mum put her arm around my shoulder to steady herself whilst I held the baby up for her to see. Was perfect! Mum had a really small second degree tear that needed a couple of sutures in. Whilst midwife I was working with did that, I did the baby check (I thought the baby had positional talipes (previously known as club foot) but wanted to tell the midwife away from the parents in case I was wrong), gave vitamin K and weighed the baby. Did tell midwife; she came and confirmed it was talipes. By this time it was an hour after my shift was meant to finish. Every day this week I have done between an hour and two hours extra each day in the hope of getting spontaneous vaginal deliveries (SVDs) and today it paid off! I got catch number eighteen! I am pooped, and it's only 8p.m. All I am fit for is sitting on the sofa with a large glass of red wine getting slowly pissed. The end to the perfect week!

Now, my standing delivery today went beautifully, but the same can't be said for one of my fellow student midwives who also experienced a standing delivery recently . . . with a somewhat different outcome. She had been poised ready to catch the baby. Mum was standing and pushing. Baby delivered a little quicker than expected and she fumbled to catch the baby but missed (eeekkk!). The baby bungeed on the cord, which snapped right at the umbilicus and the baby proceeded to haemorrhage, needed transferring to NICU. Baby was OK, but student midwife was rather frightened by the whole experience! Oops!

Sunday

Had a wonderful day off yesterday. The sun came out and I just pottered about in the garden. Was a really relaxing day. Got up at 6a.m. this morning, and was at work by 7a.m. Sat in coffee room waiting for handover (7.30a.m.) and listened in horror to the shift from hell the night staff had just had. The unit had been closed again because they were full (second time in a week), there were women in every room, most high risk, meaning they required one-to-one care. Was in for a busy shift.

My mentor and I were allocated the care of two first time mums, both thought to be in early labour. They both needed assessing. I took one, she took the other. My lady had mild and irregular contractions. Popped her on CTG and got a beautiful trace for thirty minutes. Contractions were becoming more regular, and because delivery suite was sooo busy again the decision was made to do a VE to check whether she was in established labour; if she wasn't she could go over to the ward. She had been given a VE at 5.30a.m. and I did another; disappointing, no change, still 2cm dilated. So warded her. Exact same thing happened with my mentor's lady, too.

Next, got given the care of another first time mum. She had come in for induction as was post dates. However, she had arrived the night before with a history of reduced fetal movement. The docs had decided to scan her and found reduced amounts of amniotic fluid and the decision was made to not give Prostin, but to ARM her. That was done in the early hours of the morning. I took over to a working epidural, but absolutely rubbish CTG trace, the baby had reduced variability for long periods (an hour and more), with no accelerations. Docs called; plan was to continue to monitor carefully because they were about to perform another emergency section, and this lady would have to wait till after. So I carried on observing things closely. Got called out of the room by the midwife in charge . . . thought I had done something wrong, but she said there was a man waiting for me! Walked down to the midwives' station and the dad from the emergency section I had done a few days ago was there with the biggest bunch of flowers you have ever seen! They are gorgeous! And a bottle of Champagne, a card, and a photo of my mentor and me cuddling their daughter. Made me cry. It's so lovely to feel appreciated! He was very complimentary towards my care, and said I would be a wonderful midwife, and could he book me for next time . . . how sweet. (This was all said in front of my mentor, and the midwife in charge!)

Anyway, back in room, trace continued to be rubbish, and I continued to get docs in to look at it. Woman in theatre was having a huge PPH (postpartum haemorrhage) that was delaying everything. Finally, at 1.30p.m. the consultant came out of theatre, came and looked at my trace and the decision was made for a crash section. Off we dashed to theatre . . . I scrubbed to catch the baby, a beautiful baby girl weighing in at around nine and a half pounds! So, first week back on delivery suite, started well, two catches on first day back, followed by two emergency sections, lots of first time mums slogging it out with epidurals and Synto, one more catch, and another emergency section. Am hoping for more catches next week. Beginning to feel like I am jinxed. Although I mustn't complain, I have learnt so much this week, and have had fantastic midwives to work with; might just pop open my Champers to celebrate how fantastic I am! Ha ha ha . . .

Week Forty-four

Monday

Worked an early today. After the chaos of the last few days I got to work to find only three women on the board. One who had delivered and was ready for transfer to the ward, one who had a section yesterday and was high risk, so still with us on delivery suite . . . and one who was slogging it out in labour (a first time mum) with an epidural, Synto and a crap CTG trace who was expected to turn into a section rather quickly. Midwife in charge asked what I would like. I said Synto lady, but mentor suggested we ward the lady who had delivered and wait to see what else came in, so that's what we did.

Took lady across to ward at 8a.m. and did some tidying up and checked controlled drugs etc. Got a lady in for assessment with a history of abdo pain and PV (per vaginam) bleeding. I did it all, was fabulous. I took her to a room, took a history, did obs, found and listened to FH, got her to do a urine sample and checked her pad, reported back to midwife in charge. Got doctor to review, assisted whilst he did a speculum examination and took an HVS (high vaginal swab), and then I did all the documentation and took her across to the ward. First time I felt like a proper midwife! What also made a difference was that there was a wonderful midwife in charge. She is very into normality, which really comes across in her approach to running the delivery suite, fantastic. She is very supportive of me and encourages me in every way to become involved, and gives me ample opportunity to learn and stretch myself (a change from the old hag yesterday whose softly-softly approach is actually a cunning cover for the back-stabbing bitch she really is).

Filled time popping some details onto the computer, then got the call saying a multip was on her way in contracting three in ten . . . sounds hopeful! As soon as she walked through the door my excitement drained away – she didn't look like she was in labour. She looked far too comfortable. I took a history; she had SROM'd the night before, and started contracting at 7a.m. this morning. I did an abdo palpation and then popped her on a CTG. Nothing was happening . . . she was contracting one in ten and was quite comfortable. Discussed this with mentor who had a chat with doc; because lady had a section previously and her waters had broken she was high risk and decision was made to speculum and take an HVS. So I did that! Then she was to be transferred to the ward for close observation.

That was my shift . . . no more deliveries . . . definitely feel jinxed. Have tomorrow off, so need to crack on with my essay and try and get it finished. Will ring round fellow student midwives and see how they have been getting on, too. Am also going to try going to the gym again, has been two whole weeks since I hurt my knees. Spoke to the physio today who agreed it was an acute gym injury, and that I needed to take things easy and not go on the treadmill, or do leg presses. She also recommended that I work out for just thirty minutes, not an hour and fifteen minutes, and that I work my way up gradually. Am going to try that, and see how I get on. Starting tonight hopefully!

Tuesday

Have not been to the gym. Have however spent the whole bloody day working on my essay, and it still isn't finished. Got to the point where I was trying to gather research evidence from the uni's digital library where nothing I wanted was available online . . . urrrggghhh! So, after searching the Internet for hours for the three vital articles I needed, I gave up, collected the kids from school and drove a forty-mile round trip to uni and back, just so I could photocopy the bloody articles in the library and carry on working on the essay tonight. Hubby was not best pleased when he got home at 5p.m. and the house was empty and no tea was on the table. Wouldn't kill him to actually make his own tea after work.

So, have now written the main body of the essay, just need to write the conclusion and pop in a couple of appendices. Will carry on with it tonight, and also have tomorrow morning and Friday morning to do a bit more because I am working lates on both those days. Had a chat with fellow student midwife (who failed her exam) today. She is still waiting for results of re-sit, having expected them by letter by now. I told her to ring uni and ask what was going on, but she is going to wait until the end of the week and see what happens. Am worried that she is falling behind with clinical experiences. She only has nine catches so far, and although she was meant to be on delivery suite all last week, she only did one shift, working the rest of the time with ladies on the antenatal ward because they were short-staffed. Tried to encourage her to get herself back on delivery suite, so I hope she does. Also chatted online to one of the others in my group; she is as stressed as me at having to write all these essays, work full-time, prepare a presentation, arrange clinical assessments, and run a house and be with hubby/kids. Just feel like I couldn't do anymore if I tried. Right, must get back to essay . . .

Thursday

Not much to say about yesterday. Looked after a lovely first time mum. She was having the typical long first labour, had an epidural and Synto IV, looked after her for the whole shift and she was still 9cm dilated when I left at 9.30p.m. Got into work this morning for the early and found out she had had a forceps delivery in the early hours of the morning. Bless her. Popped to say congratulations.

Was hoping my luck was going to change today! The board didn't look good in handover (was a quiet shift . . . just first time mums in early labour). Was allocated the care of the most advanced first time mum . . . fully dilated! She had an epidural and Synto running, so we got her pushing. After an hour the CTG was dodgy with late decelerations, so doctor was called and he decided to do a Neville Barnes Forceps Delivery (NBFD). Baby was born within minutes after that, and a big baby he was too, over 10lb! Whilst I did the immediate post-delivery care we were allocated the care of a multip (hip hip hooray!) and I was sent to assess her.

Now, this looked promising . . . two previous babies, contracting three in ten, requesting pain relief but didn't want Entonox. Did a VE and she was 4-5cm dilated, so Meptid was given. She quite happily laboured for the next hour and I popped in and out. She buzzed for me at one point, saying the contractions were feeling stronger and lower . . . This was my prompt to get the delivery set open, draw up the Syntometrine and get my gloves ready (have learnt that much by now!). Stayed with her during the next contraction and she felt pressure in her bottom. Called mentor who did a quick VE and she was now 8-9cm dilated . . . good, good! Mentor left, and with next contraction she gave one almighty push and vertex was visible! Buzzed for mentor to come back again. Got gloves on, and the baby's head delivered. Cord loosely around the neck, which I was able to lift over baby's head easily; next push and the baby was out! A catch . . . at last! The poor baby had a congested face (blue/purple colour), but was well and happy.

Went for lunch, and saw I had a text from fellow student midwife who is waiting for her exam results . . . letter should have arrived today but didn't. Looked at my mobile just as I was about to do my clinical assessment and she had sent me a text saying that she had failed, although she only knew unofficially. Did my assessment in a panic, worrying about her. I passed it (thankfully). Went back to delivery suite and shift was finishing so they sent me home (five minutes early – a definite first!) Changed out of my (blood splattered) scrubs and dashed to the car.

Phoned fellow student, but she had someone with her.

Got home and spoke to her straightaway. She had found out that she had failed from personal tutor who had rung to offer her support after receiving her letter; only problem was she hadn't received the letter, so she found out for definite that she had failed just because of this phone call for support. Apparently they are now offering her an oral exam. Had previously been told that we had only two attempts at anything and would then be asked to leave, so don't know quite what's going on. My heart goes out to her. To get halfway through the course and then be asked to leave would be awful.

Had an incident with son this afternoon, too. He has been so good, and really been playing nicely with a couple of other boys his age. He asked to go to the park with them, just around the corner. Normally I wouldn't allow it, but this time I thought I would give him the benefit of the doubt. Just as tea was ready, twenty minutes later, he came flying in through the door, sobbing his heart out. One of the older boys (who had been at the same childminder as him until we parted ways, and had always bullied him then) had started hitting and kicking him, pinched his bike and threw sticks at him. Hubby went round to the park and told the boys off, saying he would contact their parents if it happened again. My lad wouldn't stop sobbing. It's so unfair. I know because of his ADHD he is a target for bullying just because of his limited social skills. But this one older boy seems intent on making him as miserable as possible. Saw this particular boy putting his middle finger up at us on the way to school the other morning in full view of his father. Incredible.

So, after having a high from my catch, I now feel absolutely rubbish again. Selfish mother (for going out to work), rubbish mother (for bringing up a son badly, and allowing him to be bullied). Just crap really. Tried to overcome these feelings and took both son and daughter to the music evening at school tonight. Hubby didn't want to come, obviously! Sat on my own, felt paranoid that everybody now avoids me because my son is the naughty one. Need to focus on how lucky I am to have two beautiful children, and be settled in a comfortable home, training to do the best job in the world!

Friday

Think I am getting depressed. Feel on the brink of tears the whole time . . . nerves are shot to hell and basically would love to just disappear with kids and never come back here ever again. Hate living in a little village with stay-at-home mums who have nothing better to do than gossip and make judgements about everyone. The looks, the whispers. It's horrible. Just want to protect my little boy from these nasty bullies. He now has a bruise on his neck and on his leg from where this older boy has been pushing him around. Am going to write to the school, and hopefully something will happen then.

Sunday

Little boy has been amazingly well-behaved over the last couple of days. We had a wonderful day out yesterday at Woburn Safari Park. Children were disappointed that the monkeys didn't jump on our car, but we got very close to tigers, lions, black bears, wolves, rhinos, zebra, giraffes and loads more . . .

Friday was a good day at work too. Got to work for handover and yet again there were no women labouring; in fact, only one woman was on the unit and she was just being sent home. Midwives offered for me to practise my venepuncture skills on them so they all lined up and I took blood from them all. No misses thankfully, was really nervous! A woman just turned up with a history of SROM, discharge and reduced fetal movements. So I took care of her, popping her on a CTG and generally checking her over. Because of her unsure history of ruptured membranes we did a speculum, but her membranes were intact and everything was normal so I sent her home.

Then we got a call from the ward. They were inducing a multip, had just done a VE and she was 4cm dilated with bulging membranes, so she was being sent across for an ARM. I was given the task of doing this; good practice, having only done a couple in the past. We were being given handover by the ward midwife and I noticed that this lady had a card stapled to the front of her notes; she was a caseload lady for another student midwife. I pointed this out rather begrudgingly. The midwife in charge grabbed the card and screwed it up popping it neatly in the bin. I was horrified! Maybe this is how I missed my caseload ladies. She was saying something along the lines of 'well, you're here and she's not, so you should be doing this'. My face must have looked as horrified as I felt, because my mentor rummaged through the bin, found the card and rang this other student and filled her in on what was happening with her lady. The other student said that she had her forty catches, and if the lady hadn't delivered by the time I went home then she would come in. So off I trotted to do an ARM. The plan was to ARM her, then nip out and have some tea whilst she established into labour and then for me to get a catch!

ARM was quite easy, thankfully. I always worry that I'll aim the sharp little hook at something very delicate and cause the lady pain, but I used my finger as a guide to feed the hook up to the bulging membranes. With a swift twisting motion I popped the bag of waters and was fleetingly splashed with warm liquor as the waters drained away. Her contractions immediately gained strength and regularity. Had to set up Entonox for her as she was in a great deal of discomfort. Nipped out to let mentor know what was happening and to get a birthing ball. Mentor was to have her tea first, then come and take over from me whilst I had something to eat. Went back into room, and within half an hour the woman was involuntarily pushing at the peak of her contractions. Called mentor back and she did a VE to check full dilatation. She had an anterior lip, which was easily pushed over the baby's head during the next contraction. I had prepared my delivery set, Syntometrine and Resuscitaire so everything was ready. Then I listened into the baby's heart rate and it had dropped to 80bpm and stayed there. We called for the midwife in charge. A push later and vertex was visible and then the baby was delivered, cord wrapped three times round her ankle (little monkey), which I wasn't expecting . . .

When I tried to lift her onto her Mum's tummy I couldn't get her there, and tugged a couple of times trying to work out what was holding her back. My mentor pointed out the cord, and clamped and cut it quickly so Mum could have a cuddle. So that was my twentieth catch! Halfway through my catches; a real milestone. Was wonderful. Poor lady (who had lost it big time somewhere between my ARM and the birth) was apologising for crying and shouting, and kept saying sorry. I gave her a big hug and told her how fantastic she was. She had been a real star.

Have pottered around the house doing jobs this morning. Nipped to the supermarket for some foundation (can't go to work without a face on!), washing, ironing, Hoovering . . . just about to make lunch and then disappear off to work for my last delivery suite shift of this stint. Fingers crossed I will get number twenty-one, would be nice!

Week Forty-five

Monday

Can you believe my luck? Got to work for the late shift yesterday and there were no women at all on delivery suite. Fantastic! Made myself a cuppa and settled in the coffee room for a good old chin-wag. Within a few minutes the phone was ringing like there was no tomorrow. Three women wanted to come in. We were allocated the care of a first time mum who had already been in that morning and been sent home in the latent phase of labour. Great . . . Woman arrived about half an hour later. She looked pretty convincing, huffing and puffing like a trooper. I admitted her, and took a history. She had SROM'd at midnight and her contractions had become stronger and more regular around midday. She was asking for pain relief. I did a VE; mentor agreed she looked like she was in active labour now. She was 4cm dilated, and the baby was OP; double great, no chance of this being a catch. First time mum, baby OP . . . Gave a shot of Meptid and spent the next few hours popping in and out of the room, giving support and listening in to the fetal heart.

At about 5.30 she asked for some more pain relief, and I did another VE to assess progress. She was now 8cm dilated, and the baby was still OP. So she had another shot of Meptid. Bless her; she managed to sleep between contractions. At this point we popped her on a CTG because her membranes had now been ruptured about seventeen hours. Managed to get out of the room and have a bite to eat. Went back in half an hour later to relieve my mentor and she really looked like she was cracking on. She was feeling all the contractions in her back, very typical with the baby in the OP position. But all of a sudden she felt pressure in her bottom and the urge to push. Now with a baby in the OP position women often get a premature urge to push, so I was trying not to get too excited. I waited for the next contraction and observed her involuntarily pushing, so called my mentor back into the room. My mentor did a quick VE to check she was fully dilated . . . she was . . . we were off . . . second stage and pushing!

She pushed like an absolute dream. Within about half an hour we saw the vertex advancing. Was itching to open my delivery set but woman was a first time mum so I held back. After another ten minutes lots of vertex was visible and delivery was imminent. Got set open, put apron and gloves on and prepared to catch a baby! Woman's partner was in awe of what she was doing; it was quite touching to share the moment with them. Baby's head delivered beautifully. Apart from compound presentation (hand was up by the baby's head) the body delivered easily too. Did the usual clamping of cord, Dad cut cord, and I popped Syntometrine in.

So I finished my two-week delivery suite placement with catch number twenty-one! Only nineteen more to get in another four-week placement at the end of the course – will worry about that nearer the time. Said my goodbyes to my mentor and she was lovely, saying she would write me a reference if I wanted her to when I applied for a job at the end of the course. Came home happy (and tired, am always tired these days).

Tuesday

Productive day! At last! Got so much done. Dropped kids off at school this morning, happy knowing that son was seeing the school nurse in an attempt to help him with his impulsive behaviour. Came home and wrote the conclusion to my complex care analysis, checked reference list, printed it, and popped it in a folder ready to hand in.

Nipped to supermarket, got son some three-quarter-length trousers for the summer, daughter a gorgeous summer top and crisps that I had gone for in the first place, and then went to my community mentor's house for lunch. She signed off all the bits in my portfolio that needed signing and we had a good natter. I told her all about my son, his ADHD, the bullying, and she surprised me and said her son had been in a similar situation. He is now doing his A-Levels, and getting on really well. I hope my little lad gets through this like hers did. Will ring the school nurse tomorrow and have a chat with her about how things went today; son seems very positive about their talk.

Anyway, so, after getting complex care analysis done, and mentor signing the bits I needed in my portfolio, came home, got kids from school, had tea, watched a fab film with the kids, chatted on the phone to fellow student midwives, although midwife who failed the exam for the second time hasn't been answering my calls. Am worried sick about her, will try calling her again tomorrow.

Have also managed to get neonatal care analysis finished, reference list checked, printed and popped in a folder. And dare I say it, have started the final of the trio of essays which are due in three weeks' time. Have every intention of finishing the blasted thing tomorrow. The plan is done, and have the guidelines/policies for the topic already. In theory, all I need to do tomorrow is find some research studies about it and write the essay. Easy!

Wednesday

Am depressed . . . know the signs and symptoms, and I must be. Have this constant feeling of gloom, my mind runs away with me always thinking about the 'what ifs' and choosing the most negative outcomes. Feel like I can't cope. Hate living in this little village now. Used to feel quite at ease here, but now I constantly get ignored by other mums, to the point that I shy away from having any contact with anyone whatsoever. Little boy is home sick today, was desperate not to go into school. Father-in-law sat with him whilst I took daughter to school, and I popped in and had a chat with his teacher. Was worried that something had happened at school that was making him not want to go, that he was in some sort of trouble, but teacher said there have been no incidents. He quite often says he is feeling unwell in the mornings as a ploy to stay at home. Makes me worry even more. Just want to cry . . . cry, cry, cry . . .

Thursday

Had a lovely day at home with little boy yesterday. Planted some tomato plants and runner-bean seeds. Picked up daughter from school and then went on a bike ride down to the next village and back – the sunshine was gorgeous! Spoke to school nurse who was very positive about her chat with him, and it sounds like the school are going to be implementing some changes . . . about time too. Also got the majority of my final essay done.

Got kids to school this morning, and daughter fell over grazing her knee and bumping her head. Think her pride was hurt more than anything. Took her into the school to get her cleaned up and then heard that my son had been hit in the face with a bag, and was having a major nose-bleed. He is prone to them, bless him, but the blood was everywhere. He said it was an accident and the boy who had done it didn't mean to. Anyway, brought him home with me, and had to ring work (my first day on the day assessment unit, typical) to say I would be in a little late. It's now 10.40a.m. and it has stopped bleeding and not re-started, so am taking him back to school and will drive straight on to work from there. Joy.

8.20p.m.

Got to work by just gone 11a.m. Was full of apologies, but they were all very accepting and understanding of what had happened this morning. Was really good on the day assessment unit (DAU). Was a bit daunted because it's all the complicated antenatal stuff that they

149

deal with, and the midwives have decades of experience, but I was pleasantly surprised. I was basically allowed to get on with things (taking bloods, doing CTGs etc.) and just checking with the midwives before allowing someone home. Felt useful, and the midwives encouraged me to think for myself rather than have everything spoon-fed; was brilliant.

Got home to tired kids, and got them off to bed as quickly as possible. Neighbours were all outside on the green in front of the house with their children. Didn't get a wave or a nod, in fact was completely ignored . . . bloody gossipy bitches, the lot of them. Have had a 'eureka' moment. Don't care what others think of my family, or me, as long as I know I am doing my best for my kids and we are all OK, that is all that matters.

Friday

Rubbish morning. Was in an antenatal clinic from 9a.m. till 2p.m. Went on for hours, and instead of being hands-on it was very much 'take a back seat and watch what's happening'. So, five hours of boredom. Got better when I went back up onto the assessment unit. Got given two ladies to sort out. Took their blood, both of them! Am a pro at this now! And referred one to the doctor, due to PV (per vaginum) bleeding.

Got home to find my little boy waiting with a huge grin on his face. He whispered to me that he now has a girlfriend and that he wants to buy her some chocolate at youth club tonight! Am so pleased at hearing something normal from him! Made my day. He also told me all about how he had been playing with his friends at break times today at school.

Plan for this evening is to try and finish off the last bit of my final essay (not the final ever, but the final of the trio that are due in three weeks' time), to drink the bottle of Champagne that was given to me a few weeks ago, and then to chill out all weekend, enjoying the sunshine, my children, my life!

Sunday

Nearly got essay finished Friday night, just need to photocopy a policy from work tomorrow and I will be able to put the finishing touches to it. Haven't done anything midwifery-related all weekend! Yippee! Pottered about in the garden yesterday with kids. Today I took the kids swimming first thing and then to the wildlife park after lunch. Hubby has been his usual grumpy self and not joined in with anything (oh joy), just ignore him now . . . think kids are used to it too . . . in fact, me and the kids have really had fun these last couple of days.

Did do something rather extravagant, am really excited! Haven't told anyone yet; hubby, with his mood, would do his nut (ooops!). Anyway, although an absolutely huge Madonna fan, I wasn't able to afford to go to see her on her last tour. Did the two tours before that ('Reinvention' and 'Drowned World') and also saw her at the West End in 'Up for Grabs' too. Well, have always had rubbish tickets, sitting a long way away from the stage and had always promised myself that next time she toured, I would be the sad cow who goes and camps outside the ticket office for front-row tickets. Really sad, I know. So, Madonna's summer tour is announced! She is only playing one night at Wembley . . . Went on to the website and tickets go on sale Friday. Can't get to London on Thursday or Friday because of work (am only on the assessment unit for two weeks, so can't really miss anytime there). but there was a link taking you to the pages where you can buy VIP tickets! So had a quick peep – was only meant to be a peep, it listed everything you would get with the VIP ticket including top price tickets from the promoter's hold, Champagne, pre- and post-show party, laminated VIP ticket, pressie . . . Oh my God, sounded so fantastic! So fantastic in fact that I bought two tickets for the grand price of nearly a grand (£930). Fuck – wanted to scream and shout and tell the world I was going to see Madonna. Didn't, it's my secret for the time being!

Week Forty-six

Monday

Woken up early by the sunshine and birds this morning. I cursed! Bloody knackered for the rest of the day . . . never mind. Walked the kids to school, skipped home, still excited about my extravagance over the weekend.

Got to the assessment unit and was surprised at the calmness of the place for a Monday morning. The two mentors I had worked with last week were both on days off, so I kind of hovered between the three midwives who were working. No-one really told me what to do, or what I could do, so I just got stuck in. Didn't make any decisions without checking with the boss first; was a bit awkward when things were quiet and I was just standing there waiting for stuff to do . . . but the day passed quite quickly. Got more practice with taking bloods (a couple I would never have attempted before, although I thought I could feel the vein I couldn't see it, so was working blind but got them both!), popping CTGs on. Women were mainly coming in due to reduced fetal movements, or they were out of area coming in for their antenatal care check-ups.

Got home and found an email from one of the girls in my group. She has taken to emailing me her essays. Don't mind, in fact am really flattered that my opinion counts to her, but just needed an evening chilling. I sent her a text to say we would chat on Wednesday when we have a uni day (seems like yonks since I had one of those). Then my mobile rang; it was one of the three-year direct entry student midwives. They have an exam coming up at the end of the month and I had lent her all of my revision notes. She feels like she will never learn everything that could be in the exam. Remember that feeling well . . . It's horrible! But then I guess it's part and parcel of the course, we all go through it.

Tuesday

Am going to see Madonna . . . am going to see Madonna! Novelty hasn't worn off yet! Told the midwives at work yesterday and they looked completely unimpressed (need converting). I think it's money well spent; I can't wait! Anyway, back on the assessment unit again today. I believe it's diabetes day – yippee – lots of large women, with large sweaty bellies. Can't wait (not). Have managed to do a load of washing, hang it out on the line, tidy up and still have time for a cuppa before I have to head out the door.

6.30p.m.

Enjoyed my day on the assessment unit. Same old stuff really, bloods, CTGs . . . Saw an amniocentesis being done too. It was quite emotional for me because I struggled with the same emotions I had experienced all those years ago (had to hold back the tears). Even started feeling useful by the end of the day, answering the phone without immediately having to ask a question or hand it to someone! Am going to try and finish this third essay off once and for all tonight . . . know that will make me feel loads better. Going to have a bath first –candles, bubbles – bliss!

Thursday

Yesterday was a waste of time. Had morning and afternoon lectures with a group of the second-year student midwives. They were all very nice, but the topic was sickle cell and thalassaemia, which as nurses we knew all about. However the lecture was very much aimed at those who had no background understanding of either, and consequently it was a very boring day.

Student midwife who failed exam only stayed till 11a.m. and then disappeared off. She has arranged some private tutoring through a recently-retired senior midwifery lecturer. Didn't really get a chance to chat to the other girls that much. Had arranged my next tattoo removal session during the lunch break, and because of road works in the city it took me an hour to get there and back, so missed time with them. We drove home together, and we are all really worried about student midwife who failed. She looks so delicate at the moment, like she could burst into tears at any moment. Think I would too if I were in the same position.

Managed to finally get the third of my trio of essays done last night. Haven't got time to look at it properly this morning as am working in the assessment unit again (10a.m. to 6p.m.), and again tomorrow (8a.m. to 4p.m.). Have managed to get Monday off though, so will use that productively and just check through the references lists, and make sure that I am 100% happy with what I am handing in. Have a few last minute ideas for the reflection, but am on the word limit (including the 10% extra we are allowed), so can't really add anything without taking bits out, and there are no bits I can take out either!

Just got back from dropping kids off at school. My neighbour, who I keep meaning to nip and have a chat with about the Madonna tickets, wasn't doing the school run today; her hubby was. Don't really want to go and knock on her door, she's probably having a lay-in. But tickets go on general sale tomorrow, so don't want her to try and get some if she's up for one of these VIP tickets I have.

7.20p.m.

Got home about forty-five minutes ago. Had tea on my own again; the others had all eaten by that time. Went and knocked on neighbour's door but she wasn't there. Work was good. Left to my own devices again really, with the midwives checking what I had written and done through the day. Had some anti-D ladies this morning; these are ladies who are rhesus negative blood types and are given an injection of anti-D immunoglobin at around twenty-eight weeks of pregnancy to help prevent complications in future pregnancies. Then a couple of reduced fetal movement ladies, and even a stretch and sweep (hope it helps get her started). Am meant to be going back into work tonight to get something signed in my portfolio, but don't have the energy. Am going to go and enjoy a nice soak in the bath instead!

Saturday

Was my last day on the assessment unit yesterday, am really going to miss it. After everyone telling me how rubbish it would be, I really truly enjoyed it. I found it challenging, with loads of learning opportunities. After a wobbly start to the day (antenatal clinic boring as hell – love community ones, but this was keep pinching-myself-to-stay-awake boring), went back up to assessment unit at lunchtime to find the place chock-a-block full. Was given two ladies to look after. Both nearly term. One had a breech baby and was opting for a vaginal delivery. She hadn't felt baby move much that day and had come in for monitoring. She was already on the CTG so I introduced myself, checked the CTG and said I would be back shortly. The other lady had raised blood pressure (BP), excess protein in her urine, headaches and facial oedema, therefore they were querying pre-eclamptic toxaemia (PET). I did her BP, was normal. Checked her urine, no protein . . . weird! Popped her onto CTG and went and picked the brains of one of the experts! Plan was to repeat BP and urinalysis after getting good CTG trace and if all OK, she could go home on the understanding that she must ring straightaway if she felt bad again. She is being induced on Sunday, so will only have a day at home. CTG was fine and I sent her off.

Breech lady's CTG was also fine. Although she was still not feeling the baby move, the CTG was picking up adequate movement. Reassured her, and discussed position of baby and placenta, but she was still very worried. Again referred to one of the experts who said she would scan this lady to check if the baby's position had changed, or if the fluid levels had decreased. Whilst I was getting her ready for the scan, I asked her if she would mind me caring for her during labour. This would be an amazing opportunity for me to see a breech vaginal delivery . . . She and her partner were more than happy for me to be there, so I gave her my mobile number. She will call when she goes into labour! Scan was fine; the baby's still breech, fluid all normal, so she went home too. Was 4p.m. by this time, so I said my thanks and goodbyes, and headed home too.

Daughter has gone on a scout camp for the weekend. Son is still asleep in bed (it's 8.30a.m.), and hubby has gone to do weekly supermarket shop; he's guaranteed to spend at least three times the amount I would, and fill the trolley with crap like beer and crisps – hate it when he does the shopping. Have popped washing in the machine, switched the dishwasher on and think I will head upstairs for a shower. House is an absolute pigsty, so have to concentrate on giving it the once-over today.

Week Forty-seven

Tuesday

Ended up going out on Saturday night with hubby, to the birthday celebration of one of my fellow students . . . a Chinese in the city! Was lovely, would have been even better if hubby hadn't been there. The mum of one of my daughter's friends babysat. Had asked her for recommendations for a babysitter, and she said she would do it! Not everyone in my village think we are the devil's cohorts. Anyway, got very drunk and had a fabulous time!

Tried to keep little boy occupied over the weekend; was hard work. Got up ready for school yesterday and he was in tears not wanting to go, saying he had no friends, that everyone was horrible to him. Went and spoke to the head teacher . . . have had enough. Son is meant to be going on a residential trip Wednesday to Friday and am so worried that he will be bullied and teased, resulting in him reacting to it and ending up doing something impulsive and silly, and then be the one getting into trouble for it. Had a good chat with the head teacher who reassured me that they were seeing now that he was being teased, and what he used to get into trouble for was his reaction to these nasty boys. Only trouble is these nasty boys' parents have all ganged up on us now . . . get awful looks from them outside school, they put their heads together and whisper and look over . . . bitches. Then to top things off, little boy comes out of school with a letter saying that before school club is closing at the end of next half-term. Am sure I am not meant to be a midwife – what am I going to do? Just feel very fragile, keep crying. Need to get signed off sick (stress and depression) but can't. Only got seven months left on this course, can't quit, can't interrupt either because this is the last ever conversion course the uni are doing. So, would have to start the three years from scratch . . . rubbish.

Have taken to walking the dog over the hills, listening to Madonna on my iPod, and just escaping from my life . . . feels free . . . love it! Got home yesterday to find a message from the family support people we have been referred to by the school paed. They are coming out on Friday to talk to me about what they can offer. They had wanted hubby to be there too, but he shows no interest in being involved in any of this, as expected.

Start a two-week stint on the postnatal ward today, although I'm meant to be focusing on antenatal ladies, work that one out! I know?! I've got three lates in a row. Sorted it purposefully that way, so I could be at home and take kids to school to see son off on the school trip tomorrow. Don't want him to go, but have to give him a chance . . . He went last year, but that was with the year above (there were some spaces, and his name got pulled out of a hat from the year below). This time it is with his own year, and all those nasty boys who bully him. Started me off again; can't stop crying.

Wednesday

Have decided that I have to be positive to stop that horrible feeling inside me. Little boy got off on his school trip this morning and I know that he is going to have an amazing time! I took the dog for a lovely long walk over the hills, listening to my iPod and sang at the top of my voice the whole way. My daughter is doing her cycling proficiency this week at school and she looked mortified when I walked past with the dog, blowing her kisses.

Work was good yesterday. Am focusing on antenatal care, so my mentor and I had the antenatal bay, with lots of different jobs to do. One lady was twenty weeks pregnant with vaginal bleeding; another was 13 days overdue and in for induction of labour (IOL); another was thirty-eight weeks pregnant and in with vaginal bleeding (she was also a drug user and scans were showing her baby was very small). The final antenatal lady had raised blood pressure and severe symphysis pubis disfunction (SPD) . . . so quite a mixture to keep me busy. Looking forward to going back in again this afternoon.

Thought I had better make a start on my dissertation. But I switched the computer on, read my emails, went on Facebook, went onto the Student Midwives Sanctuary, just checked the uni website in case the results of my research essay had been posted (they haven't, am hoping it will be Friday) . . . and now, should really attempt to start dissertation.

Thursday

Got into a routine now; school run, long walk with dog! Love it. Have been making myself think positively about son being away. Miss him to bits, but am still hoping he is having an amazing time!

Work was same old, same old . . . bit boring actually. Did the antenatal bay again. Lots of inductions of labour, i.e. putting Prostin in – lovely. Have worked with a different mentor everyday this week, and although it's nice to see how people work and do things differently, it's also pants because they don't know what I can and can't do. So end up doing not a lot really. Can't really concentrate on it this week what with everything else.

Looks like the friend I wanted to go to the Madonna concert with can't afford the tickets, so am going to have to ask around . . . my bank balance is appalling at the moment! Ooops.

Sunday

Don't know where to start. Son came home from school trip; teacher assured me he had been well-behaved! Rang a friend on the off-chance she would want to go and see Madonna, and she jumped at the chance! And will pay me all the money for the ticket next week, so won't even have to use the credit card I have applied for (that was worrying me a lot).

Popped over to give fellow student midwife, the one who failed her exam, her fortieth birthday pressie on Friday. She is very delicate; her oral exam is coming up on Wednesday . . . tried to encourage her best I could . . . must be an awful situation to be in, though. Only saving grace is she actually finds out on the day whether she has passed or failed (so, whether she is still on the course, or being chucked off). I am doing a late on Wednesday; will keep my mobile in my scrubs pocket.

Weather has been miserable today. Hasn't stopped raining. Took son to supermarket to get him a cheap PlayStation game for being good whilst away with the school. Came home, watched *Britain's Got Talent* (recorded from last night). Took kids to drop off birthday cards to my little bro, then drove to other little bro's house to drop off the Indiana Jones DVD we had watched the night before. Fab film . . . (have got the new Narnia one to watch tonight).

We all thought that on Friday, we would get the results of that rubbish research critique it took me forever to write. Nothing was posted onto the online message board, and surprise surprise, the bloody exam office wasn't answering the phone, so we have been left in limbo over the weekend. Bloody typical of the uni, they can't organise anything – useless! I mean, they have given us a very strict timetable of when the bloody essays have to be handed in, but we haven't a clue when they will be marked, or when we will get the results. Sums them up actually . . . rubbish. And the only decent lecturer out of the lot has retired. Least we only have seven months left. Feel sorry for the three-year girls.

Week Forty-eight

Tuesday

Got to uni, dreading a whole day of smoking cessation lectures. Had only been there an hour when my mobile rang. As an excuse to leave the room I went and answered it. Would normally leave it . . . glad I didn't! It was delivery suite. My breech lady had been admitted and was 4cm dilated. Perfect opportunity to leave what was going to be a very boring day! Trying to hide the wide grin on my face I apologised to the lecturer and the other girls and left.

Got to delivery suite about an hour later after driving very fast down the motorway, and popping home en route to get my portfolio folders and work shoes first. She was now 6cm dilated and had an epidural in situ, although it wasn't working well. I took over her care. After about an hour it was evident that the epidural was really not doing its job, so I called the anaesthetist to re-site it. This was done, and immediately she was pain-free! Popped the urinary catheter in, and spent the next couple of hours giving top-ups, listening to the fetal heart, taking observations and keeping the paperwork up to date. Senior midwife I was working with was very pro-normality and she ensured the doctors, all chomping at the bit to get involved, were kept at arm's reach! I did a VE four hours after the last one; was very strange feeling a squidgy little bottom under my fingertips instead of a hard head. Another two hours later, she was fully dilated. Due to the fact that the baby was breech and she had an epidural, we waited an hour before pushing commenced. Then she started, and boy did she do well. As a first time mum, with an epidural, it was questionable that she was going to do well, but she pushed and pushed, and baby's bottom was visible very quickly. By this point the doctors were outside the door, hovering in the corridor. The baby's bottom was on the perineum and she pushed it out with ease! I had to pop my fingers under baby's legs and kind of flick them out, but they both came easily (doctors were now in the room behind the curtain!). My mentor whispered in my ear to check the cord. I did, and it was pulsating. Next push delivered more of the body and I twisted baby from side to side and unhooked the arms. (Doctors were now in aprons standing behind me!) Cord was twice around the baby's neck, but loosely. Baby was all out apart from the head, and it seemed like an eternity before the next contraction came (doctors now had gloves on too but I didn't budge from my position). Then my mentor told me to pop two fingers under the perineum and flex the head, to aid delivery. This worked and baby popped out immediately, followed by the placenta. Baby was flat, so I clamped and cut the cord, and mentor took the baby to Resuscitaire where the paediatrician was waiting. Baby just needed a bit of facial oxygen and soon pinked up and was introduced to Mum!

So, I did it! I delivered a term breech baby! Was amazing! Definitely one I would like to reflect on in an essay . . . will have to write my next reflection about that! I need to learn all the names for the manoeuvres my mentor had talked me through. Got home, knackered but happy and thought I'd check my emails quickly. Don't know why, but also looked at uni's message board. Results for the research critique were there. I passed! Got a 'B'! (Relieved that I had passed, but bloody disappointed that I had not got an 'A' – stupid, I know!). But it's a pass; I did it! I let the other girls know the results were there.

Wednesday

Oh my God! Don't know where to start . . . Fellow student midwife re-took her exam for the third time today, it was an oral version this time. Anyway, she rang me at 11a.m. to say she had passed! Am pleased to bits for her . . . can't lie; she had us all worried that she wasn't going to make it. But she's done it!

Got to work for a late shift and took handover on the ward. Had just done one postnatal check when the senior midwife from delivery suite came across and said she was going to have to pinch me, delivery was heaving, and she needed me as a senior student to come over and care for a lady. The word 'fuck' was being slowly repeated over and over in my head, but off I trotted, a lamb to the slaughter . . .

On delivery suite I was told to take over in room five. As I entered, the mum-to-be (first time mum) was having an abdominal palpation by another very senior midwife. When this was finished, the midwife asked me to pop the lady onto a CTG because her abdomen was only measuring 30cm at 3 days overdue (very small) . . . rather worrying. So nipped out to get CTG. Took it back into the room and the midwife handed me the notes and said get on with it. 'Fuck fuck fuck' was now being shouted inside my head . . . Keep it cool, keep it calm . . .

Set up CTG whilst the lady's boyfriend and mother watched me, am sure they could see me shaking, then tried to reassure her. After about half an hour she asked for pain relief. I have had a ticking off for giving someone Entonox without a midwife's say-so, so off I trotted to get the OK for Entonox . . . got the OK and set her up with it, and she used it brilliantly. Thought I saw a couple of fetal decelerations, so I called senior midwife into the room. She was happy with CTG trace and reassured me. Felt stupid . . . felt really stupid, and I apologised to her outside the room. She said don't be silly, she would prefer it if I called her when I was concerned rather than try and cope alone. Entonox began to lose its effect, as the contractions got stronger and my lady was asking for something more. So I checked with the senior midwife and then did a VE. She was 5cm dilated, with bulging membranes, and when I told her this it seemed to reassure her and she decided not to have any more pain relief. So she carried on using the Entonox, puffing away like a real trooper. Her membranes spontaneously ruptured.

An hour and a half later she started pushing. I tried to get her to breathe through the contractions but she couldn't. So reluctantly (hoping I wasn't going to be red-faced again) I pulled the call bell to summon the senior midwife. I updated her, and she hovered in the background watching through the next couple of contractions. At this point I saw the presenting part! She was bloody doing it! And quickly! The senior midwife went to get the Resuscitaire, and Syntometrine, and I opened my delivery pack and got my gloves ready. My lady kept pushing and pushing. The senior midwife whispered to me that I was going to lead the delivery and she stood back watching from by the door. (Didn't have time for the 'fuck fuck fuck' bit inside my head this time, I had to concentrate!). So, I led the delivery, encouraging her to push when it was the right time and telling her when to pant. Her gorgeous little girl was delivered very quickly, and was perfect! I finished off, tidied up the room and left to check the placenta whilst they had a cuddle.

Checked placenta in the sluice, then went off to get some vitamin K for the baby. Passed midwives' station and the senior midwife in charge called me over, pulling out a seat next to her and patting it. ('God, I'm in for it now,' was what I was thinking; 'must have forgotten something and she was going to embarrass me in front of everyone!'). So I sat down, preparing myself for the ritual put-down-the-student-midwife to begin, and looked round at her. Rather alarmingly she had a huge smile on her face, put her arm round my shoulder and told me how well I had done and how she was testing my abilities by giving me that lady to care for. She went on to say that I had managed the delivery perfectly, and that she was really pleased with the care I had provided! Couldn't believe it! Nearly burst into tears, I was so relieved. I told her that when the lady had started to push involuntarily I was worried that she was pushing onto cervix because her baby was OP; pushing prematurely was quite common with an OP presentation, and that's why I had wanted to VE at that point. She smiled, and said it was a justified thought process, but that with experience I would know. So she sent me back off to the room with the vitamin K to do the baby check and carry on. On the way back up the corridor, an MCA called me into one of the rooms as I passed. She said she had heard what the senior midwife had said and that I should be very proud, because this particular senior midwife rarely gives praise. Wanted to cry again; what's wrong with me? Am so hormonal lately! Better not be pregnant . . . well, no chance of that. You have to have sex to get pregnant . . .

Thought I might be sent back to the ward at this point, but no.

Instead I was given the care of a twenty-two weeker with hyperemesis (basically, continual vomiting). Did her admission, and got docs to assess her. Her urine indicated lack of food and fluids, and she was admitted to the ward for IV fluids and antiemetics. Piece of cake after my last lady!

So, there we go . . . got catch twenty-three! Rather unexpectedly! Am on an early tomorrow, is now 11p.m. so must get off to bed, as alarm will be waking me up at 6a.m. tomorrow. It's summative assessment day too. Big meeting with mentor and tutor, so am hoping that I pass. Am buggered if I don't, because portfolio is due in on Monday, and I won't have time to arrange another summative if I fail! Tutor said not to worry, that I would be fine. Hope so!

Thursday

Am on that roller coaster again. Ups and downs . . . Yesterday am up, today am down. Worked really hard on the ward. Was doing it all myself and really enjoying it. Focused on postnatal checks (mums and babies), did drugs, bloods, liaised with doctors. Cared for a cute little baby who had an extra digit on each hand. Was odd; hadn't come across that before, but had read all about it. This baby's toes were also fused together. The mum was saying it ran in the family and she had been expecting it. Another little baby had an odd cord stump. The vessels seemed to have haemorrhaged and the stump looked like a little balloon filled with blood. The paeds checked it and said it was OK. Mentor I worked with was fabulous and let me get on with it all; she just kept a watchful eye on what I was doing.

Had an early lunch and handed over to the late shift. My mentor and I sat down ready for my summative with my tutor. We waited and waited and waited . . . She didn't bloody turn up. Wanted to grab hold of her and give her a good shake, was absolutely fuming. Had gone to so much trouble to arrange the assessment on the day she had requested. My two main mentors were both working nights, and I had arranged to work a week with a new mentor, requested that we worked this particular shift on this particular day, and she forgot all about it. AAARRRGGGHHH! So, rang and left messages for tutor on her office phone, her mobile, rang the other tutors; no-one was answering. I have my portfolio due in on Monday and no-one was helping me . . . left work feeling like shit. Sat in car ready to drive home and my mobile rang; it was her. Felt like cutting her off and not speaking to her, but answered and asked her outright where she was. We had been waiting. My tutor admitted she had forgotten! Fabulous. She said she was on her way to the other Trust to do another student's assessment and that she had forgotten about mine. My tutor couldn't do it tomorrow because she is doing one with the student midwife who failed, failed then passed her exam (who has been given an extension so why she is a priority, I don't know) and she is miles away on a study day on Monday when the portfolio actually has to go in. She said to hand it in without her signatures and she would make sure it was OK. Likely story, like I can trust what she says. I just feel so mad with her. It might not be important to her, but it is to me. If I fail the portfolio it means I can only achieve a 40% mark, so all the work I have put into those three essays I have just written will be for nothing. Why the student midwife who also had her assessment booked for this afternoon didn't say anything to me, I don't know. She knew my assessment was today . . .

Have emailed my cohort leader to get her opinion on what I can do. It's not my fault my personal tutor never showed, so if they try and mark me down for it I will be really pissed off. So instead of having a nice Friday morning with my kids I have to ring around the uni and get the nod from someone high up that this won't affect my marks. Am going to kill her next time I see her . . . will end up in prison and will never become a midwife!

I sent texts to the others in my group and none of them have replied . . . just wanted a chat and cheering up I guess. Did have a missed call from one of the three-year girls who started a few months after me. She has her exam tomorrow and is really nervous. Spent half hour chatting to her. She is very clever and I know she will do fabulously in the exam, but those pre-exam feelings are horrid. I remember it well. She said she will let me know how she got on when she is finished tomorrow.

Am going to go and snuggle up in bed, watch the TV, hopefully have a good night's sleep and forget about my stressful week at work. Makes a change not to be stressing about my son, so I guess I can't complain. He has been so well-behaved this week. Have promised to take them swimming on Saturday. Weather has been rubbish so we haven't been able to spend any time outside. Had a corker of a thunderstorm the other night. Was lying in bed waiting for my little boy to come and give me a cuddle because the thunder was so loud and the lightening so bright, but he slept through it! Daughter was on a sleepover at a friend's in a tent in the back garden and got drenched! She thought it was a huge adventure though!

Week Forty-nine

Tuesday

Fabulous weekend, if you ignore the jerk of a husband I had the misfortune to marry. Took the kids to Alton Towers on Sunday, hubby refused to come. It was sooo much fun. Took ages to get there and it was a bit drizzly for the first hour or two, but it was worth it! Both my kids love big fast rides, so we went on everything together. My daughter and I were hanging on for dear life with our eyes shut tight, whilst my son was pretending to be Superman with his arms stretched out in front of him! Mad! We bought the DVD of us on all the rides. The day cost a fortune, but we came home very happy, and very tired!

Uni was good yesterday. Lovely to see everyone back together again, including the 'passed on the third go' gal! It was deadline day for the three essays and our portfolios, so didn't dare look at them again, just signed them into the box. Will be six weeks before I know the results, so need to try and forget about it for a while.

We had the lecturer who normally has us in fits of giggles, but we have worked out now that she is the only one out of all of them who really gives a shit, so I have a lot of respect for her. Just ashamed that it took me so long to realise this. She was organising our alternative placements, which is where we go to one of the other Trusts covered by the uni and spend three weeks experiencing midwifery elsewhere. I am the only one going to this particular Trust, and I asked if it was possible to spend as much time on delivery suite as possible, because it feels like we don't have long enough there (over the whole eighteen months). The lecturer said I will be the only one out in practice that month so I can spend the whole three weeks on delivery suite! Excellent! Can't wait to get out there and do it now!

Have had a bit of a hoo-ha about my elective placement. The Trust near my aunt and uncle have offered me two weeks, which is what I needed to arrange. But the logistics of being away from home for two weeks is too much, so have accepted one week and arranged to go back to the day assessment unit for the other week. But the DAU is within my local area, and the uni are saying that I need to go out of area to complete this placement. They argue that it is because I need to prove my negotiation and organising skills; haven't I done that? Anyway, my argument is that any extra time spent on DAU is fantastic, because it is all high-risk care, and I learnt so much whilst I was there. Have emailed my own personal tutor about it and have just got to wait and see what she says.

Yesterday afternoon was spent re-visiting suturing, and we got to practise suturing a perineum on a piece of grey sponge! Not at all realistic, but was good to practise again, I had completely forgotten all of it from the last lecture. Have just written myself a reminder to refer back to as needed!

So, today . . . miserable weather . . . rain, rain and more rain! Switched on computer to start prepping for my dissertation and the keyboard wasn't working. Checked all the connections and couldn't get it to work, so rang hubby. He had no idea, so packed bag and drove the twenty miles to uni – was actually time well spent. Was able to start my literature search and use the uni's printer and ink to print off loads of articles. Stopped off at the supermarket on the way home and bought a large lever-arch folder and A-Z dividers. When I got home, I put all the articles I had printed into the folder, in alphabetical order . That way I won't be shuffling through mountains of paper every time I need to find a particular article.

Stopped and had a break and collected kids from school. My little lad has invited his girlfriend over to play and for tea! He is on his best behaviour!

Thursday

Got an email back from my personal tutor about my elective. She is going to check with the cohort leader and let me know if it's OK to stay within area for one of the two weeks. I had also requested to meet her to discuss my dissertation, and her reply said something along the lines of 'it's too early to start worrying about that now!' I don't think so!

Have had an email back from the Trust I want to go to for my elective placement. It has all been confirmed and I even have my shifts arranged! Must ring my aunt and let her know what nights I need a bed. Need to sort out the finer details, like parking permits (a must when parking in NHS car parks), uniforms and exactly where I need to turn up and what time!

Spent yesterday in the library at uni printing all the articles I thought might be useful for my dissertation. Now have a huge folder, full to bursting! Typed out a reference list for all the articles too, and a reference list of all the articles I still need to find. Was hoping to get into the library today whilst I was at uni, but we were finished by 1p.m. and the others all wanted to head home. We share lifts, so I couldn't stay. When we got back to mine we sat and chatted for about an hour!

One of the girls was missing today. Her mum has recently been diagnosed with ovarian cancer and she has had to travel back home (overseas) as her mum has taken a turn for the worse. Was awful without her. Nobody knows when she will be back. She has just gone indefinitely . . . I would do the same in her position, but I know how much she wanted to do this course, and I just hope that she does come back.

Walked down and collected the children from school. Still have that daily battle with trying to make eye contact with the other mums, most of whom still avoid me due to my naughty son. Have accepted that they are the ignorant ones, and that I am doing everything I can to support him through trying to manage his behaviour. In fact, the family support people are coming tomorrow at midday for our first session on controlling techniques. Am pleased, and nervous, and a bit miffed that I could really be doing with spending the day in the library prepping for my dissertation. Don't have many more private study days now, will be working full-time and the two weeks annual leave I do have will be spent with the children because they will be on their summer holidays. Help!

Am going to look on the Internet for a nice campsite to take the children to for the last week of the summer holidays. Will need a holiday by then – need one now, but will definitely need one by then!

Friday

Ordered seventeen articles from the MIDIRS (Midwives Information and Resource Service) website last night. Cost me £30, but spent most of the evening searching online for the articles and couldn't get full text versions of them. I know some of them I can get from the library, so I didn't order those ones. Will photocopy them myself when I am at uni on Monday.

Have had an email back from the cohort leader about my elective. She wants me to do two weeks out of area. Have told her this is not possible, so will just have to see what she says. Am refusing to bend over backwards for this university. They are bloody useless. We went to collect our essays from the exams office yesterday to find that the office was closed. When we managed to get hold of someone, we were told our essays were on a different campus (100 miles away) and that we would have to request for them to be dispatched to our own campus so we could collect them. Bloody ridiculous! So, I emailed the exams office and have requested they be returned to our campus for Tuesday next week, which is when we are next there. Haven't had a reply yet . . . won't hold my breath.

Anyway, had better get on with doing some reading . . . dissertation hell here I come! OK, it's now 3p.m. I have to do the school run in ten minutes and what have I achieved today? Sweet F.A. as far as my dissertation is concerned. I did have a helpful meeting with the family support people, and have been introduced to the 1-2-3 Magic programme, which I am going to try out on my kids tonight. Sounds amazing; just need to see if I can do it! Drove up to the stationery warehouse and bought a new academic diary, seeing as mine is due to run out within the next four weeks. My life is in my diary, so that was a big priority. Still have my dissertation stuff in front of me. Now have three reference lists; number one is articles in my folder already, number two is articles I still need to get from the library, number three is articles I have ordered from MIDIRS. Just need to read them all now. Am going to start on that tonight, and can then indicate on my reference lists which articles are research, discussion or just commentary. Sounds simple enough . . .

Week Fifty (OMG!)

Monday

Uni today; the timetable had the instructions 'bring a banana and an unused teabag' so was quite looking forward to finding out what on earth we were going to be doing. Got to uni and only one of the girls was there. One was sorting out her portfolio; she had got an extension due to failing the exam, and was handing it in a week late. One was seeing her mum onto a plane, who was flying home after a week's visit.

One was still overseas with her poorly mum – no news from her yet.

So, we sat and chatted for a bit, the lecturer told us that the eighteen-month conversion course we are on, supposedly the last one the uni was running, is now being re-introduced next year. They have funding for fifteen places. Those 'in the know' have realised that with the huge amount of midwives retiring over the next five to ten years, there will not be enough newly-qualified staff to cope, so there is now a huge push towards recruiting! One of the girls I did my nursing training with was desperate to get on the course with me, but the uni lost her application form. So I told her straightaway . . . she is really excited, and told me she had already spoken to the uni and is considering applying although she is in a job she loves, and is worried about leaving. Sounds like me when I was having to hand my notice in for my job before starting.

Finally started talking about multiple birth (which was on the timetable for the morning) but was boring . . . Managed to resist the temptations of the tuck van at break time, and sat in the sunshine with a cup of tea. The three-year girls who are about to qualify were there. They had had their OSCEs (objective structured clinical examinations) the week before and had got the results. Loads failed. Sounded awful. We heard all about it. Am very scared. After break, we sat and talked about care in labour of a woman expecting twins . . . was actually really interesting and I was surprised to find it was 12.30p.m. when I looked at the clock. We had a short lunch break before the 'banana and teabag' session. During the break I rang the exams office. They said that they could not find our essays or our integrating study proposals. They don't know their arse from their elbow.

Anyway, back to bananas and teabags. We were having a lecture by an ODP (operating department practitioner) about epidurals and spinals . . . what's the connection? I know; that's what we were thinking. So, it got to the point where he said we could practise doing an epidural (the anaesthetist would always do this, it is never the role of the midwife, but as midwives we support women through the procedure and therefore need knowledge in regards to what it is, what it does, drugs etc. as we would be topping them up). He gave us all a 500ml

171

bag of fluid. On top of this we put the teabag; on top of the teabag we put the banana. Then we taped it all in place. Next he gave us all an epidural pack. The plan was to site the epidural in the banana (stay with me now). Pushing the epidural needle through the banana skin was like pushing the needle through human skin . . . slight pressure required then pop – it goes through. Next, we connected the air-filled syringe (would be filled with saline in practice). Pushing the plunger very gently in short bursts, the needle was inserted further and further into the banana, until the pressure was suddenly gone and the needle was in the epidural space. In reality, it was through the skin on the other side of the banana and into the teabag. Now, if you stopped pushing at that point, the needle was correctly sited and all was swell and dandy. If you continued to push, then the needle went straight through the teabag into the bag of fluid and you got wet feet! Was actually a very clever way of illustrating how the anaesthetist knows they are in the right place for the epidural, and ensuring we grasped how important it was for us as midwives to keep ladies still during this very delicate procedure.

The last bit of the lecture was about diet and fluid in labour, and was same old same old. Cohort leader popped in and said that I had to go out of area for my elective placement, although going to one of the uni's other Trusts was OK. The Trust which is OK is the one I worked for as a scrub nurse! Rang them when I got home and spoke to my old boss, explained the situation and she is happy for me to go back and work there as a student midwife for a week. Means I get to see everyone again, have a laugh, and do a job I loved! A win-win situation, I believe!

Am very conscious of the amount of time my dissertation is going to take. Don't seem to be able to get organised with reading all the research I have collected. Don't have time either . . . being at uni all day, then having family at home in the evenings. Think I need to write myself out a proper timetable to try and keep on top of everything. Although, saying that, the two weeks I have arranged to go away for my elective covers weekends, so I can work on it both those weeks during the day while the kids are at school, and the following week I

will be on leave and the kids will be at school. So that's three weeks
. . . will take longer than that though, am gonna have to pull my finger
out.

Tuesday

What a waste of a day. Uni was more than crap, it was Crap with a
capital 'C'. We all met up at my house, and instead of flying out of
the door in a rush to get to uni, we sat and had a cuppa, leaving fifteen
minutes later than normal. Got to uni five minutes late and lecturer
had flounced off in a mood to get coffee, locking us out of the room,
and not returning for half an hour. Fabulous start. Then we had to sit
and listen to her moan about timekeeping like we were all children.
So we all sat and sulked. Got our own back though; she was struggling
to set-up her PowerPoint presentation, and refused to take our advice,
adamant that she was doing it right. She wasn't, and when she finally
did take our advice her presentation magically appeared. We all sat
there grinning like Cheshire cats!

Now, this particular lecturer is renowned for promising to finish
very early if we just have a half-hour lunch, and then always finishes
late anyway. She did it to us yesterday without even asking, so today
we were all prepared to refuse. As if on cue, she said 'Right then, back
here in twenty minutes, OK?' and walked out the room. We sat in
stunned silence, all assertiveness draining out of our bodies. So, what
do children do? They rebel, of course . . . we went clothes shopping,
took about forty-five minutes, bought lunch and took it back to the
room with us! That showed her! (Childish we know, but made us feel
better!) It was at this point that she announced she was the marker
of our portfolios and essays which have just been submitted. Ooops!

Rest of the afternoon was even crappier than the morning. Only
saving grace was that incredibly she finished an hour early, so I was
home by 4p.m. Was able to enjoy a lovely afternoon/evening with my
mum. We walked the kids (and dog) over the fields and chatted. Was
nice to see her.

Wednesday

Wanted to throw the alarm clock across the room when it woke me up this morning. Three days in a row . . . rubbish, thought this uni lark was the easy option. This morning, finally, was a morning well spent. We were lectured by our cohort leader, who we haven't had for ages. Made a lovely change. She knows her stuff, teaches in an interesting way, and doesn't bullshit us when we ask a question and she doesn't know the answer. She was teaching us all about the abnormal pelvis, and OP presentation. The only moment of weakness came on our part when she left the room to get something. I put the model pelvis on one of the girls' heads and took a photo whilst she pulled a silly face. I then pretend to give birth to the model fetus, and used two fetuses as earrings by wrapping the placentas round my head.

Had a two-hour lunch break. Got loads more articles printed off in the library. My personal tutor was giving the afternoon lecture. It was the first time I had seen her since she didn't turn up for my summative assessment. Delayed making eye contact, but she was her usual self. Can't deny she gives a damn good lecture, so this afternoon was good too. It was all about the midwife's role in Caesarean sections. Have really had pangs of longing to return to my old job recently, and I can't wait to go back for a week and do it again. Seems like forever since I last scrubbed for a section, or since I recovered a lady without being in student mode. Will be so nice to just get on with a fabulous job again.

After the lecture, I had a quick chat with my tutor about my dissertation. She thinks I have chosen a subject that is too straightforward, and that I have made it difficult for myself to get a good mark because of this. I argue that a previous student did the same topic and got an 'A', and although I am tempted to read her work, I am not going to because I want my work to be my work and not influenced by what she chose to focus on. However, it proves that the subject can be done, and can be done well. Anyway, have arranged to see her again in a month, by which time she expects the majority of the dissertation to be completed. Time will tell . . .

Thursday

Didn't get to sleep till gone midnight last night . . . it was so humid, just couldn't get comfy in the heat. So was knackered before I even got to uni.

Arrived at uni on time, after a hairy drive (not a good passenger but particularly rubbish passenger when one particular student midwife is driving!). Had really thought that we had agreed that lecture would start at 10a.m. but luckily the others disagreed. Thankfully she was there and ready when we got there at 9a.m. The whole day was about grief and bereavement. Very hard going. We were shown a video about women who had experienced stillbirths, IUD (intra-uterine deaths) or late miscarriages. The lecturer had to stop it after twenty minutes . . . all four of us were crying . . . sobbing our hearts out with tears rolling down our cheeks. Had panda eyes thanks to mascara running (waste of time buying so-called waterproof mascara) . . . we all looked a right state walking into the canteen for coffee!

The rest of the day continued in the same vein. Felt thoroughly depressed by the time I was in the car on the way home. It's really hard, but the Trust I work in doesn't allow students to care for women experiencing IUDs or late miscarriages, but does expect newly-qualified midwives to care for these women. So, I know I will be shoved in a room at some point and expected to get on with it, without having had the opportunity to practise under the watchful eye of a mentor. The girls working in the Trust I will go to for my alternative placement do have the chance to look after these women, so I am going to have to try and get my experience in when I spend my three weeks up there. Daughter is hovering, waiting to get on computer. She leaves primary school in six weeks and some of the parents are putting together a memory book for each child to have a copy of. We have found loads of old photos, which she wants to scan and email to her friend's mum, so they can be included in this book.

Friday

None of us wanted to be at uni today, was just one of those days. Hubby was working from home, which meant he could take the kids to school, so I left for uni an hour early to get away from him, and in the hope I would get a parking space. Got to uni and the bloody car park was empty. Lecturer later told us we were the only students in uni that day, all the other cohorts were out on placement!

Lecture was good, but we were all in a weird mood. This was not good. Poor lecturer. She was trying to explain necrotising endocolitis to us, by drawing pictures. Not good at all . . . One of the girls burst out laughing, and her laugh was so infectious we were all laughing to the point of crying within ten seconds flat. Lecturer turned around to see us all pissing ourselves; would have been awkward had we been able to say anything, but none of us could. One of the girls finally managed to ask her what the green bit was, to which we were all on the floor laughing hysterically!

Left at lunchtime, as had another family support meeting about my son. Was good; they are teaching me how to use the 1-2-3 Magic discipline technique and so far so good. Seem to have regained some control over him.

Saturday

Apart from feeling desperately guilty that I have not done any of my dissertation yet (STILL!) I had a wonderful day with my children. Hubby was working away, was bliss! We went for a bike ride, pottered about in the house and the garden, did homework and housework and were just weekend-lazy all day. The end of the perfect day was all snuggling up on the sofa to watch *Doctor Who* (yummy!) . . .

Sunday

Hubby home today . . . says it all . . . day was shit.

Week Fifty-one

Monday

Had the long trek to city campus today . . . Really hate the journey. Have to leave an hour and fifteen minutes before lectures start and that means paying childcare costs for someone to look after my kids whilst I am stuck in a traffic jam . . . pants.

Had a lecture on sexually-transmitted diseases from 9 till 10.30a.m. Lecturer was really good and knew her stuff. She explained everything well and linked it to pregnancy, so it was useful for us. Saw lots of dodgy photos of incredibly painful-looking penises and vaginas . . . glad I have never had anything worse than thrush after seeing how horrendous herpes etc. can be. We had our coffee break from 10.30 till 11a.m. then private study from 11 till 12, and lunch from 12 till 1 . . . So basically we had to fill from 10.30a.m. till 1p.m.

We had all been given login names for a special computer programme, and had been told we would be doing some sort of exam that afternoon. None of us had ever heard of this programme, so after coffee we trooped off to investigate. We all logged in to discover that it was a nursing calculations package. Started the programme . . . it was telling us what the difference between a tablet and a capsule was, how to read a drugs chart and what different size syringes looked like. Very helpful indeed to a newbie student nurse or student midwife, but we were four experienced nurses . . . Went and sunbathed on the grass outside.

At 1p.m. we all reluctantly headed back to the computer room for our exam. Took longer to login than it did to answer the thirty questions. Was very basic stuff. Finished it, and the lecturer said to logout and then log back in and I could see my result. She said it had a 100% pass mark, anything less was deemed a fail. So, logged back in to check my result. 98%??? It showed me which question I had answered incorrectly, so I looked at it with the lecturer. I had worked out the calculation in a different way to the package, although the drug dose and method chosen were both correct. Was sooo pissed off. Lecturer just shrugged and said it was no big deal, but I do get very competitive.

Tuesday

Spent the whole day sitting and listening to utter drivel. The lecturer had no PowerPoint presentation or handouts for us, she just sat and chatted. Now, she is a hugely experienced midwife, and in-between the drivel she did say some worthwhile things. The tiring thing was listening to it all and picking out these useful snippets from the rest of the drivel that was spurting in our direction. We all got bored, very quickly. Bored student midwives turn into bitchy, stroppy student midwives . . . and boy, did we get bitchy. She drivelled on till 4p.m. By this point we were all desperate to escape. Was a relief to walk out of the door at the end of it . . .

Wednesday

Yippee! Have an unexpected day off. One of the lecturers is sick and our morning lecture has been cancelled. We had self-study for the afternoon so means we get to stay at home! Now, I know I keep saying it, but I am going to start my dissertation. I have completed the literature search, compiled a folder full of research articles, bought books, ordered articles from MIDIRS and now I am going to start. I have banned myself from Facebook and MSN Messenger until at least 9p.m. tonight, therefore I have no excuses but to sit and get on with it.

Thursday

Got loads of my dissertation done yesterday – well, wrote the introduction and planned what the subsections of the main body are going to be. Counted up the number of references I have – over seventy so far, which is bloody good I think! Wasn't such a productive day unfortunately today. Dropped kids off at school, and then was tempted by the sunshine and took dog for a long walk over the fields. Was lovely, felt really good for doing it! Tried to settle and do some more of my dissertation, but it didn't work. Those dreaded distraction and avoidance techniques I know so well were calling my name. Made the fatal mistake of checking my emails, which led to me logging onto Facebook. Enough said . . . that was it then for four hours. Can you believe that I can spend so much time on there? Read all my messages, looked at all my friends' new photos, sent photos to my friends. One went to an ex-boyfriend by mistake, oops! I sent a message straightaway saying I hadn't meant to send the message to him, and he replied! Then starting flirting . . . was quite nice, haven't been flirted with in a while! So with Facebook on and in full swing, I then logged into MSN Messenger too. That was it as far as dissertation was concerned. Then spent the next hour chatting with fellow student midwife about how guilty we felt about not spending the time writing our dissertations, but neither of us logged off! Ha ha ha . . .

In the end I had so much open on my computer that the bloody thing crashed, so I went outside and radically pruned a rose bush next to my front garden path. It looked beautiful, but was so overgrown – cut half the thing off! Looks much nicer now though. Still has lots of flowers on it, too. Daughter came out of school having been dumped by her boyfriend. This one lasted two days, but she had obviously been crying. Oh to be eleven again! Her hormones are well and truly kicking in. She threw a full-blown strop when her brother kept staring at her!

Friday

Morning lecture was interesting. Was about placental abruption, so could relate what was being said to practice after my experience with one of my caseload ladies. Unfortunately it was over all too quickly and I was heading home by twelve. One of my fellow student midwives came in for lunch, and we sat and watched some birth videos on YouTube. Whilst we were doing that the phone rang; it was the headmistress from kids' school, ringing to tell me that my son had called a little girl 'four-eyes'. Why she felt she needed to ring me I don't know . . . useless school. As a matter of fact, my little boy often tells me this particular girl tells him how horrible he is and excludes him from playtime games. Perhaps if I went into school and complained, the school would phone up her mother. Anyway, instead of getting more work done on my dissertation, I sat and watched these videos. Only got half an hour now till kids finish school so will try and do a bit more. (All the three-year girls who finish in about six weeks got their dissertation results today. They all passed, with grades ranging from 41% to 82%!)

Week Fifty-two

Monday

Crap weekend. Argued a lot with hubby. Had a lovely time away from him at school fete, my mum visited, and kids and I went to nephew's birthday party, so that bit was good!

Uni today was good. Had the one and only fabulous lecturer who really knows her stuff. Learnt about PPH (postpartum haemorrhages) and then breech deliveries. Was home by 4p.m. Kids were being good, and looking forward to going to the Speedway with Cubs/Scouts for the evening.

Tuesday

Got to uni this morning hoping for a pleasant surprise (had drivel lecturer so we weren't holding our breath). Got there on time, and room was empty. Happened to pass drivel lecturer in the corridor, who announced (with a smug grin on her face), that we would be teaching the new three-year girls the mechanism of labour. Fabulous. We were meant to be learning about emergency breech delivery, but instead spent two hours explaining the mechanism of labour to other students. Couldn't remember most of it, but in the end it all came back, and we didn't do too badly.

Wednesday

Saw daughter off this morning on the secondary school bus; she was chosen to take part in a technology competition there. Bus is due back any moment so am sure I will get to hear all about it soon.

Dropped son off at school (after having headmistress talk to me again after school yesterday about his behaviour; was dreading collecting him today but no teachers came and spoke to me . . . such a relief!). Drove up to uni to find the car park chock-a-block full. Squeezed into the last space right in a corner and got into lecture five minutes late. Lecture was about shoulder dystocia, and was actually really interesting. We did all the theory before coffee, and then had a go at managing it ourselves. They have a mannequin woman (from umbilicus to thighs), with very life-like genitalia. The lecturer positioned the baby with the head delivered, and then held onto the baby inside the abdomen so it wouldn't budge, making us practise shoulder dystocia in a simulated environment. It was fab; we all had a couple of goes . . . wasn't as bad as I thought it would be. Just need to sit down and remember all the manoeuvres that are used . . . Rubins, Woodscrew, McRoberts. So felt really positive about life in general. Same couldn't be said for failed-exam-twice fellow student midwife. She didn't grasp the manoeuvres that quickly and lecturer was very short with her and not at all encouraging. Felt embarrassed to be there actually, was very awkward. She was picked on about everything, in fact she just melted under the pressure, and it went from bad to worse.

Do have to say though that a real emphasis is already being placed on the dreaded OSCEs. We have been told that the practical stations will be video-recorded, and the VIVA (oral examination) station will be audio-recorded . . . on top of that, we have a written station. Am crapping my pants.

Had private study for the afternoon, so after finally managing to get my car out of the space I parked in this morning without hitting the Jag parked next to me (with the help of two of the girls, and a lot of patience), I came home and worked on my dissertation for a couple of hours. Think that's the way to do it, spend a couple of hours every day working on it. Have still only written the introduction and half the literature review, but then again I am very critical of what I write, and it takes me a long time. Once it's written I don't go back and do it again. It's finished, none of this first draft, second draft rubbish. Have written about 600 words, and have 2 full pages of references already! That's what takes the time! Will do some more tonight, after I have cooked tea and walked the dog. Got text from failed-exam-twice fellow student midwife; she had been called into delivery suite for one of her caseload ladies . . . fingers crossed she gets a lovely catch to make up for what she endured this morning. Poor thing.

Thursday

She did get a lovely catch yesterday, little boy at 5.06p.m.

First lecture, due to start at 10a.m. was a rep, talking to us about sutures. Got really excited – reps normally have loads of freebies, but this one was crap. Talked to us for an hour about sutures, then let us practise suturing on some fake skin slabs, then gave us a pen each and buggered off. Waste of time.

Did some work in the library. Afternoon lecture was quite interesting. It was about infertility. Only lasted till three, so was home by

3.30p.m. Kids were just walking home with sister-in-law as I pulled up on the drive, perfect timing!

Friday

Finances are bad, couldn't speak to hubby about it all last night. Knew it would all end in a row. So have waited, and tried to calm down about the whole situation. Went to uni this morning, felt like absolute crap, which my colleagues and lecturer kindly told me I looked like when they set eyes on me. Was planning to leave at lunchtime, just couldn't cope with sitting there . . . Lecturer kind of got the idea that none of us were really interested, so she finished by 12.30p.m. and we all went our separate ways.

Am now feeling the pressure from everywhere. Have dissertation to write. Kids will be breaking up on their summer holidays soon. We have no money at all (and won't for a long time), son's behaviour is still an issue. Why do I deserve to have such a shitty life?

Week Fifty-three

Monday

It's elective week and I'm not doing my hours till Friday, Saturday and Sunday, so had planned to get on with my dissertation. That was till the friend I am going to Madonna concert with dropped out (she was meant to be giving me £250 quid today towards her ticket). So decided I would try and sell tickets back to people I bought them from. After two hours waiting in a queue on the phone I gave up and emailed them. They emailed me back to say it wasn't possible to do that . . . I'll sort it. So, am going to have to work pretty hard on my dissertation tonight to make up for all the faffing around I have done. Have got it planned what I want to do. Am going to put each research paper I have on birth plans into a summary grid, which I can use to compare them.

Tuesday

Just re-read the last few days' entries and they don't really reflect the huge torment I have been through. After realising that the finances were so bad again I was in turmoil; had always said I would leave him if he got in this mess again and now I don't trust him, and I think that trust is the very foundation of a relationship, so it basically says it all . . . no trust no relationship. If I left I would not be able to provide my kids with a stable life (house, money etc.). I would have to quit my course, and then not have the financial stability to look forward to that midwifery could provide. Basically, it's my mum's life repeating itself. She stayed in an unhappy marriage till my youngest brother was old enough to move out, and then their relationship was over. Looks like I am heading exactly the same way. So, have decided to carry on, stay put, and make do. The dissertation is the last thing on my mind now, but I have to try and make myself write it . . .

Thursday

Was my birthday yesterday. Hubby didn't get me a pressie, didn't even get one from the kids for me. Wanker. So, was heading for what I thought was going to be a miserable day, but then fellow student midwife who failed her exam twice came over. We went for a long walk over the fields and talked things through. Then she took me for lunch, it was lovely. Made my day.

Went to bed early, was about 9.30p.m. The phone rang. It was my mum's partner saying not to worry, but Mum's in hospital with a suspected bleed on the brain. Not to worry? How could I not worry? Three hours later in the early hours of the morning, my brothers and

I arrived at my mum's ready to go to the hospital first thing in the morning. She was stable. The following morning we went in to see her. She looked frail and tired, but all the tests had been normal, and the urgent scan was being downgraded to an outpatients scan. She was discharged by lunch and we all took her home. Made my way home that evening and went straight to bed.

Friday

Back in theatres for my elective placement today! Was amazing. As usual they were under-staffed. My old manager said 'You'll be OK scrubbing in theatre, won't you?' I just smiled and said 'Bring it on!' So we were off, first elective section was due to maternal gestational diabetes and hypertension. Was done and dusted within the hour. Cleaned theatre, gulped down a cup of water and was ready for number two. This one was being done for breech presentation and previous emergency section abroad. Was complicated, and went on for hours. Twice, the registrar had to call the consultant into theatre, first time because he couldn't find the midline of the rectus sheath and second time because the bladder was very high, his uterine incision was very low and he was having difficulty suturing the uterus closed. Eventually the uterus was closed, but then they had to open the second theatre for an emergency section. Surgeon's assistant de-scrubbed and left to go to theatre two whilst the consultant scrubbed to finish off our complicated one in theatre one. Then . . . (yes, it gets worse) they had major problems in theatre two and the consultant left us and went to help. This left the surgeon and me . . . I was now surgeon's assistant and scrub nurse! Sent my runner to inform the theatre co-ordinator, who came in, asked if I was OK and then left (I had said I was OK and that I would call him back if anything happened). So by this time it was gone 1p.m. I was starving hungry, thirsty, had backache and we still had one more section to do after finishing this one and cleaning theatre. Luckily, the third case was straightforward and we finished by 3p.m. Needed to sit down by that point, not used to standing in theatre for hours on end! We didn't have anything else for the rest of the day. I arrived home tired, but happy!

Saturday

Second day in theatre. No cases at all . . . must be a first! They had done five sections through the night, so no work was left for us on the day shift. One of the section ladies from the night had complained of a swelling, stiff neck whilst in recovery. After having an obstetric review she was diagnosed with surgical emphysema caused by the Entonox and a possible pneumothorax. After a chest and neck X-ray, the pneumothorax was confirmed and a diagnosis of Hammonds was given. Never heard of it, so must look that one up. As I was scrub for theatre I didn't look after her, but I did sit and cuddle her baby for an hour so she could sleep.

Sunday

Arrived to be greeted by a woman being pushed into theatre for an instrumental. They managed to deliver the baby by ventouse quite quickly, so we were back in the office eating breakfast by 9a.m. They warned us of a couple of possibles, but it stayed quiet for the morning. A grumpy midwife came round about 12.30p.m. and grunted at us that her twins lady would be in theatre within the hour for an emergency section. I popped into theatre and made sure that everything was ready and then we waited for them to bring her round. I love scrubbing for twins . . . it always amazes me that one baby comes out followed by another! The procedure went well, quite straightforward and two gorgeous little baby boys arrived in the world. They both weighed around 5lb each!

After that we sat and chatted, and did some weekend cleaning. Around 7p.m. they said they had another section for us. They brought the lady round to have her spinal sited. Now, this lady was having a section for maternal request . . . big ethical issue . . . not sure that I agree with women choosing major surgery over a vaginal birth . . . midwifery is all about normality after all. Anyway, she was labouring like a trooper, and was already 5cms dilated. She was very demanding and just wouldn't sit still. Sorry, that's a very nurse-like thing to say, obviously she was in labour and therefore in a great deal of pain. The anaesthetist couldn't get the spinal in, and I had scrubbed and had my set laid out ready for the best part of forty-five minutes when they decided to give her a GA (general anaesthetic). The night staff were just coming on duty so, after checking my set with the scrub nurse taking over, I left them to it.

All done; my three days back in theatre was over before I knew it. I drove home with mixed feelings. I had been offered my old job back . . . Should I finish my course? Should I go back? I love that job. But do I love it more than being a midwife? Lots to think through.

Week Fifty-four

Monday

After seeing my daughter off on the school bus for her induction day at secondary school and taking my son to school, I have worked on my essay all day. I have decided to do a literature review as part of the dissertation, reading and summarising all the research studies I have collated about birth plans and putting basic info into a grid to enable ease of comparison. Reviewed fourteen studies . . . took me all day, but feel like I have finally started!

Tuesday

Same day as yesterday, really. Kids to school, walked dog over the fields in the rain . . . love the smell of wet grass! Back home and continued work on my literature review. Haven't got as many done today. Am up to nineteen now; sounds rubbish, but had some complicated ones to try and work out! Have just got back from a parents' evening at the secondary school and dropped daughter off at Scouts, been on another long walk with the dog, it's 8.30p.m. and am going to try and get a good couple of hours of work in now, here goes . . .

Thursday

Saw tutor this morning, and showed her the work I have done on my dissertation. Bit disappointed really, she said what I had done was fantastic, but didn't offer any constructive criticism on how I could make it better. Maybe that's a good thing?

Am off on my elective tonight. Driving down south after I have given the kids their tea. Not really looking forward to it, but least it gets me out the house and away from hubby for a few days. Will miss the kids though . . .

Sunday

Am back! Drive down on Thursday was fine. Got up early and made my way to the hospital for a long day shift on the delivery suite. Walking into the hospital I had those awful first-day nerves! But I needn't have worried. Everyone was really nice . . . they showed me where to change into scrubs and then sat me in the coffee room with a nice cuppa.

They don't have handover for all the staff on duty, just the midwife in charge so we all waited until the work had been allocated. I was working with a deputy sister and we were given the elective section list to do! Typical! So I watched two sections being done basically the same as we do things.

After lunch I was working with a different midwife and we were caring for a multip who was fully dilated and ready to start pushing. Within an hour, she pushed a huge baby boy into the world (4.950kg! 10lb 15oz in English). The unit's policy is to have a second midwife in the room as the baby is delivered (their rationale being so the first midwife can concentrate on Mum, and second midwife can give Syntometrine and catch the baby). Took a little while to do the paperwork and transfer her to the ward, so by the time we had done that it was the end of the shift.

On Saturday I was working on the ward. Absolute chaos is the only way I can describe it! Again, handover was rather strange. The midwives coming on duty took individual handovers from the night staff and then updated the others on the day shift . . . Basically, this meant that no-one really knew what was going on! The day didn't get much better. They were inundated with postnatal women, there weren't enough midwives and everyone was running round, with no real order to what needed doing . . . Wasn't much fun!

Today I was working with the community midwives. The day started badly, as there had been a maternal death over night. I realise that this caused a great deal of grief, upset and worry. The midwives who had cared for her antenatally were manically trying to find her notes, to ensure that they had documented everything . . . covering their own backs basically but who can blame them? I went off to a home delivery with another midwife. We spent half an hour with the lady; she was contracting, but only irregularly. On VE she was 3cm dilated, and coping well, so the midwife said we would leave her and she was to call if her waters broke or the pain got too much. When we got outside she said she was going home for lunch as there was no other work, and that I could go home! I had only been working for three hours! She gave me vague directions to get back to the hospital and then drove off! So there I am in a large city I don't know, no clue really where I was, with no TomTom . . . Eventually made it back to the hospital, and gave the day up as a bad job and went back to my Nan's.

Left for home at 3p.m. Was so nice to see the kids when I got back. Things are really bad at home, don't bother wearing my wedding ring anymore; sums things up really. We took our little dog for a walk and chatted about the last few days. I am spending all this coming week on my dissertation, and really hope to get the bulk of it done; now the literature review is done it should be easier.

Week Fifty-five

Tuesday

Got loads done on my dissertation yesterday . . . worked on it from 9.30a.m. till 3p.m. whilst the kids were at school. Am up to 1600 words now! Have still got today and Wednesday, Thursday and Friday this week to work on it, and Monday and Tuesday next week, then the kids are off on their summer holidays, so will be harder. Am taking them to the seaside for four days next week, near my mum's, and she has said I can use her laptop to carry on working on it during the evenings whilst we are there. After that I am back at uni for a week, then working for three weeks. We do have a reading week the week before its submission, but am praying that it is finished by then!

Life at home is pants. Well, with hubby anyway . . . am going to tell him tonight that I want a divorce. Tried to last night but it wasn't the right time. Guess it never will be, and I can't carry on living like this, so tonight is the night!

5.30p.m.

Hooray! Got loads more done today . . . am up to 2600 words, and have scanned in three more appendices, added loads of new references too! Finally seem to really be getting into it, and haven't been easily distracted by the usual eBay and Facebook avoidance tactics!

Thursday

I did it. After drinking half a bottle of red wine, I told hubby I wanted a divorce last night. Didn't go so well.

I haven't done any of my dissertation. Have spent the morning ringing round and trying to find out what (if any) benefits I may be able to claim to help me pay the bills. Have never lived on my own before, and I know I will have the kids with me but am still really scared . . . but oddly it's mixed with excitement too! Chatted for an hour to one of the girls on my course who is a single mum, and she gave me lots of advice on ways to save money and how to cope. Also rang my solicitor and have booked an appointment to see her next week to draw up the divorce papers.

Week Fifty-seven

Friday

Haven't had the opportunity to write in my journal over the last two weeks. Don't quite know what words to use to describe the immense emotional trauma I have suffered, it has been horrendous. In a nutshell . . . I told hubby I want a divorce, he was angry, and then said he was sorry and could I take him back. After a few days I told him it was too late, he had done this before and I still wanted a divorce.

Trying to work out how I will cope with the bills has been difficult, but looks manageable if I am sensible. I had decided to quit the course and become a stay-at-home mum, to give the kids the support they will need and because childcare would be impossible if I continued to work, but all my friends and family have been fantastic, talking things through and offering practical help where available . . . so I am still here, I am still a student midwife!

Uni was a disaster this week. Monday the lecturer went to the

191

wrong campus, and couldn't be arsed to then drive to us. Wednesday she was in a foul mood and snapped at us all day. Yesterday she finished by midday (we should have been there till 4p.m.). All the lecturers who are allocated to give us support on writing our dissertation are on holiday for the next three weeks, and it goes in a week after they return . . . rubbish. Have worked more on my dissertation and am up to about 4000 words now, but don't know if it's right or any good because of the lack of support from uni . . . just got to plod on and hope for the best I guess.

Week Fifty-eight

Wednesday

Did the first of my night shifts in sister Trust last night. Was dreading it, they have a crap reputation, and was fearing the worst but I actually had a really good time! The midwife I worked with was lovely, although she spent half the night slagging off the Trust I work for. Anyway, this is what I got up to . . .

On delivery suite, only three women on the board; we were allocated a woman whose baby was due in four days' time and had come in with a vaginal bleed. CTG was good, and she wasn't contracting. Got docs to review and they did a speculum and decided to keep her in over-night for observations. We had just transferred her to the ward when another lady came in; she was expecting her second baby and thought she was in labour. She was contracting five in ten. She didn't want me to do a VE because I'm a student, so midwife did one instead and she was 7cm dilated. We popped her onto the CTG because her baby's heart rate was a little high (uncomplicated fetal tachycardia), but we soon noticed some late decelerations appearing, so the docs were called. Another VE was done and she was fully dilated, but she wouldn't push! She just point-blank refused to. No-one could understand why, and I was trying to encourage her to push and explain what was happening but it was to no avail. Docs decided to do a ventouse, and we got her into the lithotomy position (legs up in stirrups), local anaesthetic was injected into her perineum and an episiotomy performed. The fetal heart rate had remained at about 60bpm for what felt like forever. All of a sudden the presenting part surged forwards and the midwife asked the doc if it turned into a normal delivery could I catch, which he agreed to. As if by magic, the head was delivered very quickly (OP position) and I just had enough time to push the doctor out of the way to catch the baby as the body plopped out too. Popped the baby onto Mum's tummy and cut cord . . . Lovely little girl, very pretty, bless her . . . Docs stayed and sutured the episiotomy, which had extended slightly on the skin only. I did all the usual bits with the baby and after Mum had breastfed and had a wash, we transferred them to the ward.

Had time for a quick cuppa, and did some checks (Resuscitaires etc.). Next we were given the care of another woman who was labouring with her second baby. She'd had a previous section at fully dilated for deep transverse arrest (where the baby's head fails to rotate in the maternal pelvis and becomes stuck). Her waters had broken. I did the VE and she was 5-6cms dilated. She soon couldn't cope with the pain of her contractions, so she opted for an epidural. By the time my shift was finished she was settled nicely with a wonderfully working epidural and just awaiting events! I was disappointed that I hadn't got a second catch that shift but ho hum. Got loads of bits in my portfolio signed off too! Drove home feeling knackered after being awake for twenty-four hours. Just got to pop son to kids' club, then will come home and sleep! I need my bed!

Thursday

Got to work and was allocated the care of a first time mum who was fully dilated and had started pushing! Fantastic! Really started to get my confidence back and I supported her through her pushing and documented all the bits I needed to. My mentor stepped back and I was in charge of the birth. The woman was amazing, and pushed like a trooper . . . within an hour I had caught her cute little girl and it seemed like the perfect delivery! I did all the postnatal checks, paperwork, transferred her to the ward and was back on delivery suite by midnight ready for the next one!

Took over the care of a lovely couple who had been planning a home birth, but she was now fifteen days overdue and had reluctantly agreed to an induction of labour. She hadn't coped with the contractions very well and had had an epidural sited, which was working perfectly. My mentor went for a break and I cared for her making sure she was comfy and monitoring contractions. The time came to do a VE and she was fully dilated! So we waited for an hour to allow descent and then got her pushing. After about an hour we still couldn't see the presenting part so the docs came to review. It was decided that she needed a trial of forceps . . . they were just going into theatre with another lady so we were asked to wait for them to be free . . . we waited and waited and waited . . . Another lady needed a crash section, but after another two hours it was our turn in theatre. Baby was delivered by forceps and Mum and Dad were both ecstatic! I did all the postnatal care and by about 6a.m. she was transferred to the ward. None of us had any breaks, and delivery suite was now empty so they sent me home early!

Friday

Had a rather eventful start to my night shift last night. Delivery suite was heaving and we (my mentor and I) were allocated the care of two women in labour. One had an epidural and therefore needed one-on-one care, the other was about 6cms dilated and also needed one-on-one care! So I was asked to care for the lady with the epidural – by myself! Was really angry and worried to begin with . . . new Trust, didn't know where things were and all the paperwork, policies and guidelines were different, but had to get on with it. My mentor went off to our other lady and I started being a midwife!

I recorded her obs, checked her epidural block, monitored the CTG and sat and got to know her, her husband and sister. Everything was fine, and after about two hours she was due for a VE. Went and got mentor, as thought I had better not do this by myself. She came in with me and I did the examination. My lady was fully dilated and I thought baby was ROA (right occipito anterior). Mentor repeated VE and agreed with me! I popped a catheter in, and the plan was to continue monitoring for one hour to allow time for baby to descend. Mentor went off to other lady and I stayed to do what needed doing. Gaining confidence every minute!

After an hour I went and got mentor and we started her pushing. She was a natural and was pushing really well. She'd been pushing for around an hour and there was still no sign of the presenting part being visible, so the docs came in to review. Baby was now direct OP and the decision was made to transfer my lady to theatre for a trial of forceps. A beautiful little girl was delivered shortly after. Again the selfish student midwife in me was angry and disappointed that I hadn't got a catch out of all my hard work . . . *c'est la vie*!

By the time we had done all that, the delivery suite was quiet again. No-one there for us to take over care of, so we popped to the ward to relieve the ward staff for their breaks. We ended up staying there for the rest of the night. It was so boring, just sitting there waiting for the shift to end. At 7a.m. they sent me home . . . But I feel it was one of those shifts that I will remember, I did provide total care to the lady I had been left with, and my mentor had said that I had done everything perfectly, and that my documentation was fabulous! Maybe I can do this midwifery lark after all!

Am glad my nights are over, not in now till Thursday and Friday next week. The plan is to do loads on my dissertation for the few days I have off, but we are telling the children about the divorce on Sunday, so guess I will have to wait and see what their reaction is, and how they are feeling. They are both booked into the summer activity camp next week, but we'll see . . .

Week Fifty-nine

Tuesday

Told the children as planned on Sunday. Felt gutted, they were both very upset and sobbed for ages. Anyway, have spoken to each of them since and explained a little more; daughter is very accepting of it all, son is more angry, but is slowly getting used to the idea. Hubby is moving out at the weekend, so things will be very different. Am worried, but only about my financial situation, am just hoping that I can cover all the bills and have enough to provide the kids with what they need.

Anyway, have been working on my dissertation. Am up to nearly 5000 words, so it seems to be going quite well. Both core lecturers are now away on holiday right through to the submission date, so can't rely on any support from them . . . typical . . . just got to crack on and do the best I can. Back on delivery suite Thursday and Friday this week (on days), so hoping for another couple of catches too!

Saturday

Phoned in sick for Thursday and Friday . . . can't believe I missed a couple of delivery suite shifts, but the pressure of the divorce was just too much. Hubby should have been moving out this weekend, but he has now delayed again, saying he might not move out after all . . . Kids don't know what the hell is going on. I wish he'd just go, and quickly.

Week Sixty

Monday

Went back to work last night and did the first of another three night shifts. Really loved it. Was very busy though; worked right through the twelve and a half hour shift with no break, and only a couple of quick gulps of water. Was allocated the bay of recovery patients to care for (with a background in obstetric recovery I could hardly refuse!). So, looked after the four post-section ladies and got them all transferred to the ward. Then I was given the never-ending job of assessments, women coming in thinking they were in labour, so I was basically giving them a thorough antenatal check, taking a history and admitting them if they were in labour (none of them were!) or sending them home if they weren't (all six!). Got a lot of practice in though, so was worthwhile. Actually got enough confidence up in the end to get on with it!

Thinking about making a nice cuppa on my walk back to delivery suite from running some notes over to the postnatal ward, I was rudely awoken from my daydreams by the howls of a woman, obviously in labour, coming from the other end of the hospital corridor. Rather absurdly, a midwife's head popped around the corner at the end of the corridor and she yelled at me to get the emergency delivery bag. Heart beating like it was going to burst I ran to delivery suite, grabbed the bag and raced towards all the noise. A fellow student midwife and her mentor were in the lift, bent over a lady in a wheelchair who was pushing for all her might. The lift doors kept trying to close, so the MCA was standing at the entrance to the lift pushing them open with her hands and feet looking like she was doing some bizarre exercise routine! There was blood and liquor dripping everywhere and an extremely frightened-looking husband sitting on the lift floor with his head in his hands, mumbling something about driving faster! The other student midwife announced that the head had been delivered while her mentor was tugging at the poor mum's trousers to try and get them off. The student midwife then announced that the baby had been delivered and was grasping awkwardly at the slippery baby in an attempt not to drop the poor little thing! I just emptied the emergency bag on the floor and passed over towels and bits as they were needed. A voice behind me made me jump. One of the paeds had also heard all the commotion, and had come to investigate too; thankfully his skills weren't needed. Once the initial chaos had calmed down, the new mum and her baby were wheeled to delivery suite. I repacked the bag that I had emptied in a panic and stood and stared at the mess that had been made. Just at that moment the cleaner arrived. Now the look on her face was priceless, wish I'd had a camera in my pocket. She looked like she didn't know whether to laugh or cry! Blood and liquor, mixed in with a bit of urine and meconium were dripping down the walls of the lift and covering the floor in the lift and corridor. Poor lady. I left her to her cleaning and headed back to delivery suite where the buzz of excitement at our unusual shift kept us going till the morning staff arrived!

Tuesday

Worked with a different midwife again last night, she was great. We had a lovely normal delivery (catch twenty-six!), and I was then allocated the care of a mum expecting her second baby, who was being induced. She wanted pain relief, so I did a VE and she was 5cm dilated. Slogged it out with her through the early hours of the morning; when I repeated the VE, she was 7cm dilated. My mentor checked the VE and said 5cm. (I didn't agree; I feel pretty good at VEs now, and was sure what I had felt). My shift finished at 7.45a.m. and she was still going strong, but not making much progress so I left.

Had to pop across to uni as had arranged to see a tutor about my dissertation. She tried to help, but didn't really. So didn't get home to bed till 10.30a.m. Have just woken up now, after sleeping right through till 4p.m. Lovely!

Wednesday

Was the last night of my run of nights and it was fabulous! Took over the care of a grande multip, this is a lady who has had more than five babies already (mad if you ask me! Hee hee hee), but she wasn't in labour, so we sent her home. Then got a first time mum who was fully dilated, and after a hard slog managed to get her to start pushing effectively. The baby's head was advancing very slowly and then baby's heartbeat dropped suddenly. We pressed the emergency bell for help and my mentor said for me to prepare to do an episiotomy. Yikes . . . not done many of these before, the thought of cutting a woman's bits makes me want to puke, but I tried to remain professional; I injected the perineum with some local anaesthetic and had the scissors poised and ready to cut, but she managed to push her baby out (catch number twenty-seven!). Did all her postnatal checks, and then my grande multip came back, in labour this time. My mentor left to get on with some other bits and I stayed to care for her.

Had been with her for about an hour and she started pushing. Called mentor back, who sauntered off to get some Syntometrine, but whilst she was gone the presenting part became visible! At this point I shit myself, and all I could think about was the trouble I'd get into if I delivered a baby without a midwife being in the room with me! Rang the call bell, and thankfully she came flying back into the room just in time to witness me catching a lovely little boy (number twenty-eight – the second of the night!!). She had a small second degree tear (along her previous episiotomy site) and mentor said I could suture it! Fabulous! A bit of practising at suturing would be fantastic, and it was a nice neat tear, so in theory simple to suture back up. But it wasn't meant to be; things then got busy again and my mentor ended up doing it herself as was much quicker than I would have been and we were needed elsewhere.

I went off to prepare the room and get the hospital notes for our next lady, who was on her way in but never arrived. We called her about an hour later, waking her up! She had gone back to sleep and her contractions had stopped. So the busy night ended quite relaxed, and I came home half an hour early.

Got home at 7.15a.m. to an empty house, rang hubby and he had decided to take kids to breakfast for a treat . . . typical that he makes an effort now, when I've filed for divorce! Am just waiting for fellow student midwife who has been working nights to pop in for a cuppa on her way home from her last night shift and then I will be off to bed for a couple of hours. Although, I have got to the point where I am past feeling tired, and I know that if I sleep too long today I won't sleep tonight, so might just stay awake all day to make sure I can sleep when I go to bed later. Bloody night shifts . . . bugger you up completely . . . would much prefer never to have to do them again!

Thursday

Spent five hours school uniform shopping for daughter, who starts secondary school in a couple of weeks. Bloody knackered now! Little boy having a sleepover in the tent in the back garden with one of his friends and they keep coming in and pestering me . . . and all I want to do (have been trying to do) is work on my dissertation – am up to 5200 words now! Have given up for the evening and am going to enjoy a glass or four of wine.

Week Sixty-one

Monday

Today was the day. Finally. Hubby moved out. Was sooo looking forward to it and when it actually happened I felt a bit guilty . . . God knows why, he brought it on himself . . . it was really strange. He said goodbye to the kids. Was tough. Felt like the biggest bitch in the world. I sent a text to my brother, he is always full of wisdom, and he replied saying that I shouldn't feel guilty, that it wasn't my doing reaching this point and that things would calm down.

Whilst all this has been going on, I have continued to write my dissertation. God knows how and I bet it will be crap, but at least I have tried. I have hit the limit of 6000 words, but have 10% extra to play with – still have one small focus to discuss, the conclusion and the abstract, so it's cutting it fine. Have a meeting tomorrow with my tutor, who is finally back from holiday, so fingers crossed she says it's OK. Little boy is going to his dad's, but daughter is coming up to uni with me.

The other thing I have started doing over the last couple of days is looking for a job for when I qualify. Whilst working in the sister Trust, they said they were advertising and I should apply . . . I know my own Trust is advertising soon, so have emailed my Supervisor of Midwives and just let her know that I am interested. It has been the bank holiday weekend though, so haven't heard back from her yet. Need to make sure my income continues, especially seeing as the situation is as it is now, although I checked my bank account today and it looks like my monthly wage has gone up by £110! That's with no unsocial hours too! Can't get too excited though, as it is going to cost £1000 a month to live in this house, and what's left has to pay for food, petrol, clothes . . . everything . . . I can do it! If I can achieve my dream of becoming a midwife then I can do this too . . . or maybe that's the half bottle of white wine I have just drunk doing the talking. Will find out in the morning!

Tuesday

Little boy stayed in my bed with me last night. He was upset that his dad wasn't there and had been crying in his own bed. He lay next to me and held my hand, bless him. Was back to his usual self by this morning. I had a really weird dream though. I was a surrogate mother for a friend of mine and she wanted to deliver the baby. I remember feeling the waves of contractions and then pushing, pushing, pushing . . . The baby's head was delivered and my friend didn't know what to do, so I was teaching her which way to hold the baby and which direction to deliver the baby in. Was really emotional. I woke up and sent her a text saying I would be a surrogate mum for her, if she chose that route.

Kids came up to uni with me when I went to see my tutor, and sat with a friend whilst I had a chat with her. She read my essay and recommended a few minor changes, but said it was fantastic! What a relief. Haven't worked on it anymore today. Son went to his dad's for an hour when we got home, and daughter went out to play with a friend, so I started painting my bedroom. It hasn't been decorated since we moved into the house seven years ago, and has cream wallpaper with small dark green flowers all over it. Have put two coats of white paint on so far, and can still see the bloody flowers. Will be worth it though, it's going to be my sanctuary . . . midwifery, husband and child-free! Yippee!

Must call my community mentor tomorrow. I start back out on a six-week community placement with her on Tuesday next week. Need to make her aware of what's been going on with me, and the fact I can't be on-call too often (although would love to be!). She is an amazing mentor, pushing me to do everything, and always asking me questions. I really like that, always being challenged. Means I can't sit back and do fuck-all, I have to be on my toes the whole time, and it's fantastic for learning. She is so experienced, and has such a fantastic perspective on midwifery – I feel so lucky to have her.

Have just finished watching *Arachnophobia* with the children, and am now jumping at any slight movement I see out of the corner of my eye! Hate spiders . . . yuk! Hope they sleep OK tonight!

Thursday

Have just finished writing the main body of my dissertation. All I have left to do is write the conclusion and a small summary and read it all checking the grammar, make sure all the references are in the reference list and typed correctly, print off three copies and get them bound and ready for handing in on Monday . . . piece of cake? Arrrggghhh! Will complete the conclusion tomorrow night once kids are in bed, and check references and read it through. That way I can print it on Saturday, and have it bound either Saturday or Sunday. Fingers crossed it all goes to plan.

Took the kids swimming today, and finished painting my bedroom. Not sure I like it after all that hard work! The walls I have painted white look fab, but I'm not keen on the pale chocolate colour I have put on the window wall, doesn't look great with the cream curtains, but I will live with it for a few weeks and see if it grows on me! It looks very modern and fresh! I found some pages of an old diary under the bed that hubby must have ripped out, and I sat and read it. It was from three years ago and basically described how I am feeling right now . . . that I was unhappy, that I was only with him for the children's sake. Made me realise that things could have gone on forever that way if I hadn't been brave enough to make the changes I have made now. Still scared about money and coping financially on my own, but I need to relax, and be careful . . . am hopeful that it will be OK.

Saturday

It's done, it's done, it's done! Have finally finished my dissertation. The conclusion is crap, but quite honestly I don't care. It's done! I spent the whole day, and a whole ink cartridge, printing it off yesterday, all seventy-one pages of it, three times over, with all twenty-nine pages of the critical literature review. The kids were so patient with me, and they came into town to get it all spiral bound with front and back covers. Refuse to look at it now; if there are any mistakes I would prefer not to know!

My community mentor rang in the afternoon. Have sorted out working with her next week, where to meet and at what times, etc. She is so kind, and we had a long chat. She was telling me she had been hearing good things about me via delivery suite, and that everyone thinks I will make a fantastic midwife! Bless her!

Kids are settling into being here with me. Daughter doesn't seem so bothered by it all, except she did mention how bad things seemed to be happening at the moment with hubby and I breaking up. We had a chat, and I think she is dealing with it OK. Son on the other hand is constantly phoning his dad, asking him if he can go down there and spend time with him. His behaviour is difficult at the moment, with constant answering back, saying stuff like 'I'm going to ring Dad, and I'm moving in with Dad when he gets a house', every time I tell him off. Think it will be easier once we are back in a routine of being at school etc. this coming week. I feel more relaxed about it all.

Sunday

Started good. Met brother for a walk with kids and dog. Came home and had lunch, then took kids to a friend's annual end of summer hols party. Got back home in time for tea at 6p.m. to find a message on answering machine from hubby. He wanted to see kids for an hour . . . They were both knackered after a busy day, needed tea, a bath and an early night as we are all getting up at 7a.m. in the morning – as I am back at uni and they are spending the day with their cousin. He doesn't realise that of course, and all of a sudden we're having an argument, with him saying 'they're my kids too' . . . blah blah blah . . . I realise they are his kids too, and I want them to spend time with him. But not like that, last minute; he knows Sunday evenings are bath evenings, getting-everything-ready-for-the-new-week evenings . . . To expect to turn up and whisk them away when they are already overtired and needing to just get to bed early is not appropriate. I rang him after kids got home, and explained all this and he apologised.

Seems like I will have to get used to this.

Week Sixty-two

Monday

Handed dissertation in today. What an amazing feeling! Am so pleased it's over. I know conclusion is crap, just hoping it's enough to get me through OK. Uni was good. Nice to catch up with the other girls. After coffee we practised handwashing, putting that day-glow cream on our hands and washing it off and checking under UV-lights . . . Was kind of cool! The afternoon in uni was a laugh. We had a breast-feeding update, which was brilliant. The lecturer is really knowledgeable, and we asked lots of questions arising from practice experiences. She has a very hands-on kind of style to teaching, and spent the whole afternoon feeling her own breasts whilst explaining positioning and hand expressing! Had a surreal moment when I looked around at my fellow student midwives and we were all sitting listening and touching our breasts . . . hee hee hee! Then she taught us hand expression on a rubber breast. It was hooked up with fake milk and we all had a go trying to express. None of us were actually much cop at it. White liquid was being squirted in every possible direction bar the cup we were trying to catch it in! Oops! It could be one of the dreaded OSCE stations, so it was nice to have a practice.

Had a lovely evening with the children. We had dinner together, watched some TV. Son popped to see his dad, and daughter tried on all her school uniform ready for her first day at secondary school tomorrow! She looked so grown-up; I had to hold back the tears!

Have just spent an hour planning the next essay (only three small ones to go now!). They don't have to be in for three months, but the sooner I get them done, the sooner I can relax and enjoy my last few months as a student midwife before the real hard work begins.

Tuesday

First day back out in community and have that terrible guilty mother feeling today that I should be at home with my children. Is daughter's first day at secondary school, and did manage to stay home and make sure she got on the bus OK. Dropped son off with sister-in-law, and made my way to a GP's surgery for an antenatal clinic.

Felt a bit out of sorts, and hadn't done an antenatal clinic for ages so was really rubbish at it. By 1p.m. we had finished, think midwife I was working with felt sorry for me (she had been through a divorce the same as me a year ago), and she sent me off home. Was lovely to be home in time to see daughter off the school bus and hear all about her first day at big school! She loved it. Hubby came for tea, but it went smoothly, he just ate and then left. Thank God.

Wednesday

Feeling much better today. Working with regular community midwife mentor. Wednesdays is her antenatal clinic day, so she got me doing all the clinic appointments and taught me how to do the computer too. Really enjoyed it. We had a couple of postnatal visits after lunch, but I was home again in time to see daughter off the bus, and we had another lovely cosy evening in together.

Got an email reply from my Supervisor of Midwives, telling me that I need to be applying for a job now! I have been online and completed the application form; I just need to spend some time writing a personal statement in support of my application. How exciting! My first job application to become a proper midwife!

Thursday

Had a quiet morning. Lots of cups of tea and chatting! Lovely . . . Did a couple of postnatal visits, and then headed to a GP surgery to set up for an afternoon parentcraft session. Had been to a couple of these before, but not really been that involved in them; this was different! We had about six couples turn up, so twelve people in all, thankfully quite a small group for my first hands-on session! My mentor led the session and spoke brilliantly, keeping their attention and making them all giggle. Then it was my turn. Oh poo, could feel my face turning that awful crimson colour, and felt myself getting hot and flustered . . . calm down, calm down! She got me to pass a bag around the room and for each person in turn to take an item from the bag. I then had to do a little teaching on each of the items! These ranged from a breast pad, a sanitary pad, a condom, a heel prick needle and a suture pack to frilly knickers (what not to bring to hospital!). It was really good, and I felt I could answer everyone's questions!

The feeding game was next, which involved two laminated cards being placed on the floor in the middle of the group. One said breast-feeding and one said bottle feeding. Each member of the group was then given three smaller cards with different things on them like 'correct temperature', 'sore nipples', 'Dad can help with feeding' and they had to choose which heading it was linked to. I led a little discussion on each card as it was put down. My mentor finished the session with a few massage techniques that she recommended for labour, and we got everyone having a practice at them! Was really good fun!

Got home by 5p.m. hungry, tired and happy! We had tea together and were all snuggled in bed by 8.30p.m. What with me being back at work, and kids being back at school, we were all exhausted!

Friday

Was told to get to clinic for 8.30a.m. this morning; I did that, then sat there till 9a.m. waiting for the midwife (not my usual mentor) to arrive, which she did in a flurry of apologies. She had lost her bag, and needed to go to the bank. Had not worked with this particular midwife before, and she asked me how far along in my training I was. I told her I qualify in four months, and she said 'Right – that's good.

You can do the clinic while I nip to the bank!' That was it. She logged me into the computer and left.

Bloody good job I had learnt how to use the computer on Wednesday is all I can say. So, my morning was spent by completing an hour's booking appointment with the first lady, followed by seeing about fifteen women for antenatal appointments. The midwife returned from the bank about halfway through the morning, to my complete relief . . . can't believe she did that! By 2p.m. I was finished and hoping to be sent home early in gratitude for all my hard work. No chance. Off we went in the car (me stuffing my sandwich down my throat with one hand, holding a fag and driving with the other). One quick post-natal visit later I was sitting in another house completing my second booking of the day, with my mentor having nipped to see another lady whilst I got on with it! Finished the booking just as she arrived back to pick me up and off we went together to complete the final visit of the day. Has been a fabulous day. I truly felt like a midwife. I had to! I had no choice but to do the job and it has really boosted my confidence, I feel like I really can do it!

Kids have youth club tonight. Son has been (from 6.45 to 8.15p.m.) and daughter is there now; as a secondary school pupil she can go to the later one (8.30 to 10.00p.m.). So that bottle of wine I have been saving for tonight hasn't been opened yet! Have managed to stop smoking again though. Not had one since Tuesday – not so much willpower as being absolutely broke, and having to keep an eye on the pennies until child maintenance is sorted out. Which reminds me, my neighbour was dropping her kids off at the before school club this morning when I took my son there. She told me she is going through the same situation as me at the moment. Separating from and divorcing her husband . . . she is even using the same solicitor as me! Have told her she is more than welcome to pop over anytime. I know how much it means just having a bolthole to run to when things get tough. Sounds like her hubby is doing the same mine did by refusing to move out and making things as tough as possible for her. Men, should all just be shot I think!

Well, here's to a lovely weekend! Oh, and I must remember to write that supporting statement for my job application.

Sunday

Have had a wonderful weekend! Went to supermarket and did the weekly shop (within budget! Yippee!). Helped little boy move his bedroom round yesterday (took most of the rest of the day). Watched *X Factor* and then *King Kong* with kids and we all crept sleepily into bed at gone 11p.m. last night.

They didn't wake up till 10 this morning. So we had a lazy morning. Spoke to fellow student midwife on the phone for about an hour. She has an extension for her dissertation and has only started writing it today (bloody bonkers if you ask me!). Gave her a few tips and tried to help best I could.

Son went to see his dad, and daughter and I took dog for a walk. By the time we were home it was lunchtime. The afternoon was spent painting son and daughter's bedrooms, and doing the gloss in my bedroom, so everyone has lovely freshly painted rooms now! Fabulous!

Have just put together my supporting statement for my job application. Have printed it and will ask my mentor to have a read of it tomorrow and tell me what she thinks. It's only very rough at the mo, still got lots more to add. Might take it up to bed with me, along with a nice cup of tea, and have another go at it.

Week Sixty-three

Monday

Mentor picked me up this morning and we went off and did a booking followed by four postnatal visits, and another booking. Sounds easy, but took us from 9a.m. till 4p.m. to get it all done (we did have an hour for lunch too, very civilised!). Am definitely starting to feel like I am a midwife though. I know I have said it a lot recently, but I now answer questions and offer information without having to look to my mentor for support. My mentor is on a late on-call tomorrow, so I'm hoping for some excitement to be called out to! Have my little brother staying over at mine, just in case I do get called out in the early hours! Fingers crossed . . .

Have been gathering research studies together for my next assignment, and also managed to work more on my supporting statement whilst doing everything in the house, managing a troublesome nine-year old and staying sane!

Tuesday

Got called out last night! I'd been asleep for about three hours and was woken up by my mobile. It was my mentor, saying that delivery suite had just called her and there was a woman pushing at home who we needed to get to quickly. She gave me the address and told me to meet her there asap. I jumped out of bed, got dressed quickly and hurtled down the stairs as quietly as you can hurtle downstairs! Grabbed my shoes, bag, car keys and TomTom and I was on my way.

Five minutes later I was arriving at the house, just as my mentor pulled up outside. She was talking on her phone and looked panicked! Had never seen her look stressed like this before. She waved for me to grab her delivery bag out of the car and we ran for the only house with lights on! Not stopping to ring the doorbell or knock, we let ourselves in and called up the stairs that we had arrived. My mentor pushed me up the stairs first and off I headed . . . Turning onto the landing I was greeted by the sight of a husband with what can only be described as the 'rabbit caught in the headlights' look on his face, kneeling on the floor behind his wife who was on all fours over the bed, with a baby in his hands! I grabbed a towel off the landing radiator and wrapped their little boy up snugly to keep him warm. My mentor was preparing the injection to help with the delivery of the placenta, and I managed to help Mum turn around (without sitting on her baby!) and clamp and cut the cord so she could have a cuddle with him!

What happened next happened so fast that I still don't know if I could ever be a real midwife. The woman started to bleed a lot, and my mentor got me to rub up another contraction whilst she prepared more drugs. The bleeding wasn't stopping so she threw me her phone and told me to call 999 whilst she prepared yet more drugs to help stop the bleeding. The bleeding eased a little, but still didn't stop. So she popped a cannula in the woman's arm and sent me with her car keys to get a bag of fluid. Oh my God . . . fluid . . . what fluid . . .where was it . . . was all in a panic. As I got to the front door I could hear the sirens of the ambulance, and I yelled at the paramedics to bring us up some fluids. Back upstairs the bleeding had settled, but the woman was now vomiting enormous quantities due to the mixture of drugs we had just given her. My mentor explained that although the bleeding had now stopped, because she had lost more than 500ml and as this was classed as a postpartum haemorrhage, we would have to transfer her into hospital anyway now.

Ten minutes later we were all in the back of the ambulance. I was cuddling her gorgeous little boy, mentor was busy writing in the notes and the paramedic was hooking up a blood pressure cuff to our woman. Her husband was following in the car behind. Because the bleeding had stopped we didn't have the sirens or blue lights on on the way to the hospital. It was a short journey, and we had arrived on delivery suite within fifteen minutes. My mentor handed over to one of the delivery suite midwives, we said our goodbyes and made our way back home to bed. It had definitely been an eventful couple of hours to say the least! It had left me wondering whether I could ever manage to deal with such a scary situation . . . Hope I never have to!

Got up two hours later, and got us all out of the house by 8.15a.m. this morning, all because I was meeting a midwife at a GP surgery at 8.30a.m. Guess what time she rolled up? 10.30a.m. I bloody sat and waited, and called her, and got delivery suite to page her . . . ridiculous! Could have had an extra hour or two in bed after last night! Anyway, was an OK day. She kept telling me to take the lead with the women we saw, but she kept talking over me and I was sidelined, so wasn't all that productive for me really. Was interesting to see how differently midwives work when they are doing the same job. Subtle things they say, the way in which booking information is given, the focus given to some things over others, the fact booking and discharge clinics are used by some and not others. I think I will take a little bit from everyone, and add my own ideas to it to become the midwife I want to be . . .

Finished my supporting information and sent my job application off last night, so fingers crossed!

Wednesday

I did my 100th antenatal clinic appointment today!!! Well, the official 100th anyway of the ones I had a chance to record in my portfolio! So no more scribbling in my folder when I am in clinic, I can just concentrate on learning and enjoying what I am doing for the last few months. I also did a postnatal visit too. Only the one though, has been an oddly quiet week as far as visits go. It was a heel prick visit, so I got to practise that, and managed to get enough blood (thank God) and not make the baby cry too much. The geographical area that my midwife covers is very deprived, I always count my blessings when I get home and really appreciate what a lovely home I have, and how fortunate I am in comparison to some of the places I visit. Have been to some appalling houses, in awful estates that I couldn't bear to live in. My heart goes out to the women and their babies, but the majority seem happy and content with what they have, so who am I to judge? My home is by no means perfect, but it's clean, we have everything we need and the area is nice (even if the other mothers from the school are all gossiping bitches).

Anyway, enough of that . . . tomorrow I am seeing Madonna! I can't wait, and have been boring everybody I have seen today with the details and how excited I am! I have got the tickets out ready. My camera battery is charging . . . I have packed my overnight bag . . . have spoken to my friend and arranged to meet her at 10a.m. so we can get the train to London!

Friday

Madonna was amazing. We had a fabulous time. Got to hotel easily. Got showered and glammed-up, and went to Wembley. Champagne on arrival, exquisite three-course meal, loads of wine . . . was wonderful! Madonna was as energetic as ever, stage was too small for the stadium though, we couldn't see the screens, but I danced the night away. Drank more in the post-show party and generally relaxed and forgot all my troubles.

Sunday

Had a lovely weekend with the kids. I haven't worried about midwifery stuff at all. Well, until I checked my email earlier and there was one from my tutor giving us the OSCE timetable for Tuesday. It's only a practice one and I haven't revised for it – and won't be doing so! After the flap to get the dissertation in, and prepping the final three essays, and working in the community full-time, how they think we have time for it all God only knows. Anyway, still not revising tonight. Might have a look at a few books tomorrow night . . . but will wait and see how I feel.

My mentor is off on leave this coming week, and I will be working with another mentor (a very senior midwife) who is lovely, but I feel quite daunted by her huge knowledge and experience, and am praying that I won't be showing myself up to be stupid. Hoping I will actually be able to work with her as daughter has a terrible headache, looks very poorly and I have just put her to bed early. Hope she sleeps it off, not like her to be ill.

Week Sixty-four

Monday

So, was meant to ring mentor at 8.15a.m. this morning, but she got in first and rang me at about 8.10a.m. There was a change of plan; we had been called in to delivery suite because there were only two midwives on duty and it was very busy! Mentor came and picked me up and we were on delivery suite half an hour later.

We had been allocated the care of a lady who was having an elective Caesarean section so I went in and completed her theatre checklist and had a chat with her. Theatre was already prepared and we took her straight through. I prepped the Resuscitaire whilst her spinal was being sited, and then I popped her urinary catheter in for her. The surgeons started, and I scrubbed to catch the baby. Everything went beautifully and she had the cutest little baby boy ever. I recovered her in the recovery bay . . . easy (was my job as a nurse after all) . . . but she decided to postpartum haemorrhage on me! Pulled the emergency bell and started rubbing up a contraction. My mentor was there instantly, and she called the consultant whilst ordering other midwives to give more drugs. The consultant decided that she needed some IV Synto so off I went to get that ready with another midwife. Drama over, she was fine, and I carried on with normal recovery care.

In the meantime, the other lady I had been allocated had delivered whilst I had been in theatre (typical). So I started the care of a first time mum who was contracting regularly and strongly. She had been given Meptid and was using Entonox to good effect. She had been 7cm dilated at around 10a.m. and it was now 1p.m. She was doing really well, with slight urges to push, but still able to breathe through them. I stayed and supported her . . . the late shift came on about 2p.m. and the senior midwife in charge ordered me off for my lunch break??? I tried to protest but just got glared at, so begrudgingly took myself off for lunch. Returning thirty minutes later I was greeted by the sounds of a crying baby from my room – yes, you've guessed, she'd delivered! Pants . . . hate the senior midwife in charge, that could have been my catch.

The community midwife had to go and do a home birth talk with a lady who had recently moved into the area, so I went along too. She was already thirty-eight weeks pregnant. I had never done one of these before, so I sat and listened as my mentor explained that the low risk criteria must be fulfilled in order for the go-ahead with a home birth. She met all the criteria and when we got in the car to drive home, my mentor asked me to ring one of the SOMs (Supervisor of Midwives) and relay all the details to her to get official approval, which I did, and she gave.

Got home feeling pleased with myself. I had coped, and hopefully not shown myself up too much! Practise OSCEs tomorrow, but am really too tired to start reading revision notes now. Am going to go upstairs and watch TV in bed.

Tuesday

OSCE day. Needed to be at uni by 9a.m. Got stuck in traffic and got there at 9.05a.m. Tutor in a foul mood, like I knew the traffic was going to be busy. I leave an hour before the start time, so not as if I don't make the effort! Talk to the hand, talk to the hand because the face ain't listening love . . . Anyway, she led us into a room with desks set out all separated in rows. Eeekkkk was like being back at school. We each took a desk. On the desk was the exam paper (face-down) and a doll and pelvis. This was the written station and we had twenty minutes to complete the question. We were off . . . the scenario was preparing for and performing an examination of the newborn . . . was helpful to have the doll in front of us, and I worked my way down from head to toes . . . one down, two to go . . .

The second station was a skills station. The scenario was along the lines of you had just delivered a baby and the woman had a vaginal wall tear which needed suturing, describe the preparation and perform the suturing. Fan-bloody-tastic! Was able to describe what I would do to prepare. Then I had to choose the instruments I needed from a box, then I had to suture a piece of foam imagining it was a vaginal wall. The suturing was appalling, I did my best, but was rubbish and I knew I had done it wrong . . . never mind, two down, one to go . . .

The third station was a VIVA (verbal) station. The scenario was that I was away on holiday when a neighbour knocked on the door and said his wife was having a baby. I described what I would do. The tutor prompted me to list the risk factors of a BBA (born before arrival to hospital) and I could only think of a couple. Felt I hadn't done very well. But managed to talk about it for fifteen minutes.

We all went for coffee and a fag and came back to the classroom for the dreaded feedback! We had all passed the written station! Only one had passed the suturing, but three of us had passed the VIVA. I had failed the suturing, but passed the VIVA, so two out of three wasn't that bad! Knew I had flunked miserably on the suturing, but hey ho.

We finished early and I picked up my son from school. He was proud because he had been given his new clarinet (I had paid for and arranged lessons before the separation, and didn't have the heart to cancel it, so will have to find the money from somewhere to pay for it all). Collected daughter from her after-school dance club and came home to make tea. Have done three lots of washing, got two lots dry, and taken daughter to Scouts. Played Othello with son, and am now preparing my portfolio for being back in the community tomorrow.

Checked my email, and there was one there about the job I applied for. Just saying if I hadn't heard anything in the next two weeks then assume I wasn't going to get an interview. Fingers crossed I do hear something, as am desperate to work in the Trust I am training in. Really need to crack on with these last three essays too, but I have no ink in my printer, and no money to buy anymore, so will have to wait till next week (reading week) when I can go into uni for the day and print off all the stuff I need for free.

Wednesday

What started off as just a sniffy nose yesterday has turned into a full-blown cold today. I didn't get much sleep last night . . . was either woken up with a blocked nose unable to breathe, or with a runny nose just pouring gunk! Lovely. Got up this morning with every intention of going to work, but within ten minutes I was shivering cold, and feeling absolutely terrible. Feel desperately guilty at taking the day off, but will stay in the warm and work on an essay, and then work clinic day (Wednesday) next week during my reading week instead. That way it's not counted as a sick day. Daughter got herself on school bus this morning, and I have just dropped son off at before school club (he still really wanted to go!). So I am back home with a cuppa preparing to write one of my final trio of essays!

Thursday

Got loads done yesterday. Planned two essays, wrote the introductions, and put in all the subheadings . . . always use the assignment guidelines and marking criteria to do that bit to ensure that I have everything covered. Just have to wait till I'm in uni to start printing off the research I need now.

Today was good. Worked in the community and did a couple of postnatal home visits and a booking, then an antenatal clinic in the afternoon. Had to refer one baby back into hospital as he had lost 200g over the 10% we class as normal post-delivery loss. Managed it all OK, and supported parents through the process. The midwife let me do it all, and was just there observing, so really feel like my skills are coming together now.

Got home to find a letter from the hospital. I have a job interview! Yippee! It's next Friday! Sent a text to friends and family to share the good news. Got lots of congratulations messages back, bless them all! Just have to get my portfolio together now, and prepare some answers to interview questions. Midwife I worked with today was telling me that for band five interviews, it's basic stuff about clinical governance, recent research and how it affects practice, where I see myself in five years' time etc. At least I have next week as a reading week so have time to prepare! How exciting! Everyone at work keeps saying I will easily get the job . . . I hope they aren't just saying that to be kind, but really mean it . . . guess I'll find out soon enough! Scary!

Friday

Definitely the end of the week. The kids were so tired when I got them up and ready for school this morning. Daughter opened the front door to see her school bus waiting on the other side of the road! I offered to take my son to school but he wanted to go in early to before school club, so dropped him off there at 8.30a.m. Least it means he likes it!

My midwife picked me up at 11, because she was on a half-day, so managed to get all the ironing done, and quickly tidied up the house (better done today than over the weekend!). We did two postnatal visits, both day five, so babies needed heel pricks doing, which I did. Then back to my village for a booking. I did that too! Mentor only had to drop some bits into hospital and then she was heading home, so because booking was round the corner from mine I have come home early. Will be able to pick up son from school . . . love doing that, it's a mummy thing I think! Have friends coming over first thing to help me move my new bed in, so will have to pop and do supermarket shop this evening. Kids will moan, but we need food!

Just been chatting to my tutor, who has been fabulous and given me lots of tips on stuff to prep for the interview. Definitely need to spend a day next week reading up on stuff like clinical governance, supervision, and the expanding role of the midwife . . . Have got so much to do! Not going to panic and get myself in a tiz. Have been to lots of interviews and I know that I do OK (as have always been offered the job – sounds big-headed, but I just seem to cope quite well in that sort of situation, God knows why!), but as my tutor said, preparation is the key . . .

Week Sixty-five

Monday

Did what I had planned to do today. Dropped son at school and then made my way to uni. Worked from 9.30a.m. till 2p.m. searching for and printing research that I need for my essay. Have got loads . . . just need to write the essay now! Plan to read through it all tonight, and then sit and write the essay tomorrow. Son is off to Cubs soon, and daughter has some homework to do, so that means I can make a good start on this one tonight. It's only 1500 words and I have done 340 on the introduction already. If I manage to get that done, the plan then is to spend the day in uni again on Wednesday searching for and collecting information for the second of my trio of final essays.

A couple of the other girls were in the library in uni too. They were doing the same as me. Didn't really get a chance to chat much, as they got there a lot later, and I needed to pop across to the maternity unit to get my mentor to sign some bits for me before I came home and collected my son from school. As I was leaving they were filling in the application form for the jobs advertised in the Trust where I have an interview on Friday; would be lovely if we all get to work together.

Really need to update my nursing and midwifery portfolio this week too. Will have to do that on Thursday. Have just written it in my diary so I don't forget. Not sure if they want to see it at interview, but at least it shows I have made the effort. Bought the posh paper when I was at the supermarket over the weekend, and ex-hubby brought round some ink cartridges for the computer today (odd), so everything I need to do it is here. Must concentrate on these essays first though.

Thursday

It's been a productive week! I have nearly finished my essay on parto-grams, just need to write the conclusion. I am already up to 1678 words (and the limit is 1650), so will need to chop out a little bit here and there, but at least the main work has been done. Also need to scan in the partograms from my own and the alternative Trusts so they are in the appendix, but that shouldn't be too hard. I thought the essay would be easy to write, and that I could do it in a day, but it has taken longer, although I am very pleased with the research critiquing, analysing and reflecting I have managed to incorporate within it, so hopefully I will get a good mark!

I also managed to print off the job specifications ready for my interview tomorrow. I have collected some information on clinical governance and supervision, and am going to spend this evening really reading it through thoroughly and preparing. Also need to do my portfolio, so can do that tonight too. One of the girls from my group is coming over this morning to walk the dogs with me, and she said we can chat about the interview, and she will ask me some questions. Have had some lovely messages on Facebook from friends and work colleagues wishing me luck. Everyone has said not to worry, that the job is mine; I hope they are right! Still can't believe I am actually in this position . . . that I have been training to do the job I always dreamed of doing, that I am nearly finished training for the job I always dreamed of doing, and that I have an interview for the job I have always dreamed of doing . . . no pressure then!

Have the wonderful task of going to have my coil checked with the nurse this morning. Have shaved the relevant bits to tidy myself up! Want to finish this conclusion before I go, so had better get on with it.

Friday

Interview day . . . stomach feels like it's not my own! Did get a good night's sleep though. Dreamt I had a delivery on delivery suite, and that I had front-row tickets to a Madonna concert! Interview isn't till 2.30p.m. so am going to go online and brush up on the Health and Safety Act. From information on job specification, it looks like they may ask me questions about it. The girl in my group who has an interview just after me is coming over this morning so we can prep together. Least I won't be panicking on my own all morning!

8p.m.

Well, don't quite know where to start – or whether what I am about to write is believable – but it bloody happened!

Fellow student midwife got here about 11a.m. We sat and had a coffee, and chatted, and we checked all our paperwork had been completed properly. She popped her passport on the table and I picked it up to have a giggle at the photo (they're always worth a good laugh!). The photo didn't look at all like her . . . She had picked up her partner's passport! Oops! Now, she lives about forty-five minutes' drive from me, so we were cutting it fine to get to her house, get back to mine and get ready to leave in plenty of time. So, we ran out the door, and drove to her house . . . got passport . . . all good so far. Then we got back in the car to drive back to mine . . . still all good so far. We got halfway back, and the car started making a really weird flapping noise. There just happened to be a police Range Rover behind us; his light went on and he pulled us over. We had a flat tyre. Now, we had fifty minutes to get back to mine, get changed and get to the hospital. So, we did what all sensible women would do in that situation. We both burst into tears! Ha ha ha . . . the poor policeman was beside himself. Through the sobs we managed to explain that we were both having an interview, needed to be there pretty darn pronto, and neither of us knew how to change a tyre. He offered to change the tyre, but failed because the nut things were on so tight. We phoned the recovery people but they couldn't get to us for an hour. I phoned my brother who was in the middle of having a tattoo done miles away. I phoned one of our fellow student midwives, who, bless her heart, dropped what she was doing and came to our rescue! The policeman escorted us to a nearby warehouse and arranged for us to leave the car outside. He must have thought we were a right pair, as we both had mascara streaks down our faces and had told him about the last time we had broken down together when her cam-belt had gone, and we hadn't managed to even open the car bonnet!

Anyway, we had been rescued. We got back to mine, in time for me to run in, get changed and run out, leaving the others with my door key so they could lock up when they were done. I got to the hospital with literally seconds to spare and sat down out of breath and shaking with nerves (and smelling of fag smoke, not good for an interview, oh well). The midwife interviewing me came to get me. I have worked with her a lot and we get on really well, so that was a good start. She asked me how my morning had been, so I told her what had just happened! We had a good old laugh about it all – it suddenly sounded so ridiculous! The other midwife interviewing was also a midwife I had worked with a lot, we had done some of my more challenging deliveries together (the placental abruption, and the vaginal breech) and I had known her for many years, as I had arranged with her to do my elective placement as a student nurse on delivery suite.

The interview questions were completely different from when I had had my nursing interview within the Trust. I have tried to remember them as much as I can, so here goes;

* What brought you to this point? (i.e. applying for this job)
* If we asked your colleagues what your three main strengths were, what would they say and why?
* Why this particular hospital?
* What do you want to achieve within your first year as a qualified midwife?
* What personalities do you find it difficult to work with and why?
* What has been your greatest achievement over the last eighteen months?
* What has been a difficult situation over the last eighteen months and how did you overcome it?
* What was your most frustrating moment during your training?
* What was the most rewarding moment in your training?

* What skills will you utilise to help your transition to being qualified?
* How will you develop as a midwife during your preceptorship year?
* Scenario one: being told by a senior midwife to do something you disagree with; how do you manage the situation?
* Scenario two: something is wrong with a patient you are caring for; how do you manage the situation?
* How do you see your practice developing?
* What sort of midwife do you want to be?
* Where do you see yourself in five years' time?
* Any questions?

And that was that! There were loads more questions, but I can't remember them all, it's already misted into a complete blur! They went through some occupational health and human resources stuff with me, and then said that I would have a letter by the end of next week letting me know the outcome of my interview . . . A whole week to wait! The midwife who came to get me saw me out, and she whispered 'Well done, that was fantastic!' and winked at me . . . so fingers crossed I will be offered the job!

I went through to the delivery suite and made myself a cup of tea, and waited for my fellow student midwife whilst she had her interview. What happened there is a story in itself, but I am knackered, have already had a glass of wine, and just need to chill out so will tell you all about that tomorrow!

Week Sixty-six

Tuesday

Have thought through what I can write about in regards to what happened on delivery suite; confidentiality is obviously paramount, so will give vague details of the scenario I found myself in after the interview last week. Basically, a couple I had cared for in the community had caused quite a stir – one was HIV positive, the other we're not sure about at this point – but the HIV positive half of the couple hadn't told the other half of the couple about the HIV and they are expecting a baby. Ethical nightmare! Could get into lengthy ethical and legal debate about this one, but don't think that's appropriate here. Will leave that one open for thought, methinks . . . The senior midwives were all discussing it and saying that it wasn't appropriate for us to break confidentiality and tell the half of the couple who didn't know about the HIV. Would definitely be an interesting one to write an essay about!

Anyway, had a boring day in uni yesterday. We were focusing on management and leadership styles, and it was very dry to say the least. Got home to a phone call from my son's headmistress about his behaviour, yet again; that put me in a downward spiral (as it always does) and I basically cried all evening/night.

Got up this morning without an ounce of motivation, but dropped son at school and waited for my mentor to pick me up. We had an antenatal clinic first thing, and were joined by a student doctor. Went really well, my mentor and student doctor checked the urines and blood pressures, did palpations and measurements, and I did all the talking and computer bits. Only had ten women, and three of them had delivered, so we had lots of cups of tea! Always a bonus!

The afternoon was spent doing two heel prick visits, and a first day postnatal visit but she wasn't home . . . will have to go back tomorrow. Then we went to a child protection meeting. Put it this way, makes you feel like what you have yourself is worth being grateful for. Very sad.

Got home to son playing beautifully with a friend from round the corner. It ended with a falling out, but he did well to play for an hour and a half nicely, outside the front of the house, instead of wandering off and getting into trouble! Daughter has Scouts tonight, and I am planning to sit and update my portfolio and then make a proper start on the second of my trio of final essays . . .

Am hoping the postman will bring me my letter confirming the result of my interview soon. They said to expect it by the middle to end of this week . . .

Thursday

Been a rubbish week as far as son's behaviour has been concerned. Can't even bring myself to write down what has been happening – it's dreadful. Gets me really down, because I do try hard to deal with it, but things just don't seem to be any better. The behavioural support lady came to see me today for a final visit. Told her what had been happening, but she said her hands were tied and they couldn't help anymore. Pants. I have written a letter to the school paediatrician asking for a further assessment, so will just have to see if that can be arranged. Just feel that if he continues getting into so much trouble now, at nearly ten years old, what's he going to be like when he's a teenager... feel like I can easily spiral into a dark helpless negative world when I dwell on it and it makes me so sad and unhappy.

Work has been good. Did clinic yesterday, a few more postnatal visits, took out some clips from a Caesarean section wound, not done that for a while! Also had a stretch and sweep to do, again haven't done that for a while either, and then the parentcraft session this afternoon. Still no letter confirming whether or not I have been offered the job, maybe I will get it tomorrow.

Friday

Didn't rush to clinic this morning. Last time I worked with this particular midwife I sat and waited for her to arrive for a good forty-five minutes. So, instead of arriving at 8.30a.m. I got there at 9a.m. She got there about 9.15, so it was the right decision as far as I was concerned! We had a quiet clinic, and she was very good at helping me talk through what I was doing as if I was in an OSCE situation. At

11.30 we had just seen the last lady when the delivery suite co-ordinator who had interviewed me last week called my mobile. She said that she knew she had promised that I would have a letter by the end of this week, but that they were waiting to receive one of my references back. I asked her which reference, and it's the one from my tutor at uni! Should have bloody known, that bloody tutor is so useless . . . she had promised me that she had sent it on the Monday before my interview. Obviously not! However, the delivery suite co-ordinator went on to say that she wanted to offer me the job! (Based on the reference being OK, and my CRB and occupational health being OK too). She just couldn't send out the official letter until the reference had come back. So there it is! I have been offered the job! YIPPEE! It still hasn't quite sunk in, I don't think. I sent a text to everyone sharing my news, and got loads of replies with congratulations messages!

We had a busy afternoon of postnatal visits, and I got home at about 5.30p.m. Have been on the phone ever since! The girl who was interviewed on the same day as me hasn't heard anything yet, although she did have a missed call on her mobile from an unknown number, but she doesn't have voicemail, so whoever it was couldn't leave a message. I tried to reassure her that the same thing that had happened to me (my reference being late) was probably what had also happened to her, but she didn't sound convinced. Bless her. I hope we do get to work together, would be fantastic!

So, am going to enjoy a glass of wine this evening to celebrate my new job. It has taken me so long to get to this point – I can't believe it is really happening! Maybe I will believe it tomorrow. My mum sent me a lovely text congratulating me on realising my ambition of becoming a midwife. I cried when I read it. I have put so much effort into getting to where I am today; it's been an uphill struggle to say the least. But I have done it! I have done it! I have done it! (Well, got to pass my dissertation, my final three essays, my OSCEs and my summative practical assessment . . . Not much more to do then! Hee hee hee . . .).

Week Sixty-seven

Monday

Had an absolutely amazing day today! Was fantastic! I worked with a different midwife because my midwife had a long weekend. She let me do everything! I did a booking first thing, then we did six postnatal visits; one included taking out beads (from a section wound) and four were day five heel prick visits – did it all! We also had a meeting at lunchtime; the new head of midwifery came to have a chat with the community team I am working with. I introduced myself and she seemed very pleasant. The postnatal visits were spread out geographically, so I didn't get home till 6p.m. but it was well worth it. I still have about twenty-five postnatal visits to document in my portfolio, and then twelve deliveries . . . and my portfolio will be complete. I can see the light at the end of the tunnel!

No news yet on my dissertation. We were hoping to have the results on Friday last week but nothing has been put on the online message board yet. But I guess I didn't expect anything less from the uni who have been consistently unreliable when it comes to results; why change now? Will just have to keep checking every day I guess.

I was under a lot of pressure whilst writing my dissertation, so am not holding out much hope of getting the 74% I need to get me a first, but I did the best I could at the time, and as long as it passes I don't care anymore.

Tuesday

Another fun and somewhat interesting day to say the least. Worked with another midwife today, as my midwife is still on her long weekend. She picked me up at about 9.45a.m. and we went off and did some postnatal visits. Nothing too difficult. We then had a clinic in the afternoon that started with two bookings. She did the first and I did the second. This was followed by an afternoon of antenatal appointments. One particularly prim and proper lady stands out in my mind . . . and will do for a long while. Antenatal bits all done, as she's leaving she tells me about her itchy hand. Alarm bells start ringing and I immediately think of cholestasis (the liver starts playing up and this causes itchiness in the hands and feet) so I bring her back in and discuss it with her, in an attempt to decide whether to take blood to check her liver function. She then very matter-of-factly tells me she masturbates three times a day (with the hand in question) and asks whether that could have caused it! Now, there's me sitting there, trying to stop myself laughing out loud with what must have been a look of pure horror on my face, with my mentor behind me coughing (trying to cover up her giggles!). Needless to say I didn't take her blood, and I washed my hands very well after she had gone! Bless her.

Wednesday

Manic clinic this morning. Only had a booking to do this afternoon, so we managed to get my final formative assessment completed after lunch. At this point I have to achieve level four, which is independent practice. I got everything at level four, which was a huge relief! I now only need one more booking, twenty-four more postnatal visits and twelve deliveries to complete my portfolio once and for all.

Week Sixty-eight

Monday

Revised for a couple of hours this morning. Mentor picked me up at 10.30a.m. and we did some postnatal visits and a booking. Feel all out of motivation – got formative OSCE on Wednesday, and know

I should be revising for it tonight, but just can't be bothered. Hopefully will feel differently about the real OSCEs.

Have got the moving bug. Want to buy my own house (never could with ex-hubby due to his bad credit history) but on a midwife's wage it's just not going to happen anytime soon. Average house price round here is £160,000. Am going to look into these part-ownership type deals; at least it's a way of getting a foot on the ladder, but with the economy the way it is at the moment, I don't even know if that will be possible.

Think I will ring the girls from my group and see whether any of them have revised . . .

Tuesday

Great day in the community. Did another two bookings (have reached and exceeded the required twenty-five), and did four postnatal visits too. In fact, we were done by 2.45p.m. even after eating lunch courtesy of a rep at the doctor's surgery! Popped into supermarket on the way home and still made it home by 3.15p.m. Hasn't given me the motivation to revise for this bloody formative OSCE tomorrow though. I have printed off some reminders on neonatal and maternal resuscitation, shoulder dystocia and hand-washing, but still really can't be arsed. Will take my textbooks up to bed with me, but am tempted to sit and read more of Harry Potter!

Am now working on Sunday instead of Friday so am going to try and get some of my next essay done, although I want to nip to town and buy my mentor a little pressie. It's my last day with her on Sunday, and I want to find her something special to say thank you to her for all the encouragement, patience, and time she has spent with me helping me through my course and sharing her knowledge with me. She mentioned the other day that she was thinking of getting herself a little handbag to carry keys and mobile in when at work; will see if I can find a nice one.

Will be glad when tomorrow is over . . .

Wednesday

I did it! I did the OSCE this morning, after no sleep and feeling really really really nervous!

The first station was written and gave a scenario of a first time mum in the second stage, head on perineum, dropping fetal heart and not wanting an episiotomy. We had to write the indications for an episiotomy and what the role of the midwife was, and then explain how we would perform one, with the rationale too.

The second was a demonstration station and was set up with a video recorder pointing at a bed with a model of a female on it from umbilicus to thighs. They gave me the scenario, which was a woman who had come in with possible rupture of membranes and we had to perform a speculum examination. I had to stand there and say my name and student number and then talk to this plastic model of a vagina explaining what I was going to do and why. I then prepared my tray and did the speculum (feeling like a complete idiot!). But it was over . . .

The third station was another demonstration, this time hand expression of breast milk. I again gave my name and student number to the camera, and started talking to this plastic boob explaining the ins and outs of hand expression, and demonstrating. Must have looked a right div, but it wasn't too bad.

The fourth station was the VIVA, an oral station where I was being tape-recorded. The scenario was being called to a woman's home who thought she was in labour, with a history of her waters breaking recently. She asked us to perform a VE and we found that she had a cord presentation. Only read about cord presentations yesterday, but could I remember anything? NO! Managed to talk through the basics, keeping fingers in vagina to ensure presenting part was not tightly compressing the cord, monitoring fetal heart, sending husband to ring 999 etc. etc. etc. Found it the hardest of all the stations, but it was the last one, so was relieved when it was over.

We all made it back into the rest station room and were told to wait for a few minutes, then one by one we could go back into the rooms and get feedback on our performances. I went into the hand expression room first. I had passed! The only thing I forgot to mention was documentation (can't bloody believe I forgot that, but never mind). Then I went into the speculum room . . . I passed that too! Had done everything right, but forgotten to offer her a sanitary pad at the end. The cord prolapse was next . . . passed that too! Had got a bit mixed up with difference between cord prolapse and presentation, but had said enough about other stuff to demonstrate safe practice.

We don't find out the result of the written station today; our papers were being taken away for marking, but three out of four so far is bloody good going seeing as I really hadn't done any proper revision!

Got home in time to pick up son from school. The whole school came out but he didn't appear, so I went in to find him. He was being told off by his teacher for apparently using a very naughty swear word . . . His teacher said his behaviour had been appalling that day. Just don't know what to do anymore. Am seeing the school doc next week, but nothing I have done seems to help. He is nine and a half, needing constant adult supervision still. I really don't know if I can carry on coping.

To top things off, one of the girls had left the OSCEs early to go for an interview this afternoon. She just sent me a text to say she didn't get the job in the Trust that she is training in – they usually look after their own. She is devastated, and is talking about packing the whole thing in. She has got it into her head that she is going to fail her dissertation, not pass these last three essays, and fail her OSCEs. She didn't get the feedback from her formative OSCEs today because she left to get to the interview on time, so I just hope she did OK in them or it will really knock her confidence. She has to wait for them to be posted out to her.

Thursday

My mentor was off today so worked with the team leader. We did a couple of visits and a booking. My nephew has a chest infection and my sister-in-law couldn't get my son from school, so I finished at 2.30p.m. to get back in time to collect son myself.

Friday

Spent the day with fellow student midwife who didn't get the job. We went into town and had coffee and cake and I tried to encourage her to continue and not quit now. She is devastated, like I would be in her position, but I think she is going to carry on . . . I hope she is going to carry on.

Sunday

Was my last day ever with my community mentor. She rang me at 8.30a.m. and arranged to pick me up at 9a.m. She had fourteen visits to do! Fantastic, I needed nine to complete the postnatal section in my portfolio. We flew around all over the place, completed all the visits by 2.30p.m. and she suggested we go and have a coffee before she dropped me back at home. She signed all the bits in my portfolio for me; it was really sad saying goodbye. I gave her a little gift box of smellies (couldn't find a bag I thought she'd like) and a card, which she seemed grateful for. We have promised to keep in touch, and I have booked her for my final summative assessment. Still can't believe that I have finished my community placement. Next time I am in the community I will be a preceptorship midwife . . . bloody hell . . . how did that happen!

Week Sixty-nine

Monday

Spent the morning working on my final reflection essay. Got 74% for both the first and second reflections I have already submitted, so I have used the second essay as a template and just gone in and changed the words to relate it to my new goal, which is suturing the perineum. Took me two hours from start to finish, just added a few different pictures in the appendix and *voilà* – finished essay! What's the point in starting an essay from scratch? It was my work originally, so I can use it again . . . guess this is a prime example of the fact that after studying and writing essays for three years through my nurse training, and then another eighteen months through my midwifery training, a total of four and a half years of study, I have finally lost my mojo and don't give a shit anymore . . . anything to finish with a pass and I will be happy.

So, I have written two of the final trio of essays, just need to print them and bind them. Only one more to go, which I have to do over the next couple of days because then the kids are on half-term holiday and I am back on delivery suite working full-time and needing to revise for my OSCEs. Should be feeling happy at what I have achieved, but actually feel bloody knackered and at the point of losing it completely. Hope this is all going to be worth it.

My community mentor rang to say thank you for the card and little pressie I gave her. She has said I can keep hold of her ALSO folder (Advanced Life Support in Obstetrics) to help me with my revision for the OSCEs . . . it has loads of stuff on the drugs and procedures to use in emergency situations so will be really useful.

Tuesday

Had appointment with solicitor first thing. She wants me to take my divorce papers to the court and sign them under oath. Weirdly I felt quite emotional about that, and haven't done it yet. Kind of took me by surprise. When I got home I spent the remainder of the day scanning all the appendices onto the two essays I have finished, and checking the reference lists. Have just printed them off and put them into their folders ready for submission. So I really have finished two of the three remaining essays!

Wednesday

Bit the bullet and went to the court this morning. Signed the papers under oath ... just have to wait for the decree absolute to come through now which my solicitor said would take about six weeks. Came home and decided to pop to the library at uni because I really can't do this next essay without a bit more research to reference.

Uni was packed with the new cohort of student nurses who started a couple of weeks ago; the car park was horrendous, but then aren't all hospital car parks? The library was jam-packed too; I had to wait to get on a computer, but managed eventually and have got the stuff I need to write the next essay. Have already written the introduction, so plan on reading the stuff I printed earlier this evening so I can start putting it all together.

The girls are coming across for an OSCEs revision day tomorrow, so won't do any of my essay, but hopefully I will do a lot of revision! That's the idea anyway, but we do tend to sit and natter when we are all together! Hee hee hee. Got a few books out of the library too, for the revision, and a doll and pelvis so we can practise the mechanism of normal labour.

Friday

Had the revision day yesterday. I didn't feel it went so well. Two of the girls got to mine about 10a.m. and we chatted about interviews (one of the girls had the interview from hell day with me and has also been offered the job, the other has an interview on Wednesday). So we helped her to prepare. The other girls arrived by midday and we got started. Within ten minutes the phone rang, it was the school asking why I was not there, the school paediatrician was waiting for me. So I dropped everything and went to the school. Was depressing listening to the details of the awful behaviour displayed by my son . . . It really got me down, and the remainder of the day I couldn't study. I tried, but my heart wasn't in it and I don't feel I learnt anything.

Son went to his martial arts club with my brother, and daughter went to school disco. I picked up an Indian take-away and we all shared it together with a couple of bottles of wine. Fellow student midwife and I had too many glasses and we were in bed feeling slightly tipsy by midnight (she couldn't drive home due to the alcohol).

Got up this morning and the countdown has started. Dissertation results day. Nerves got the better of me and I puffed away like a chimney with endless cups of tea waiting for 12.30p.m. Fellow student midwife shit herself (literally, bless her; she couldn't decide whether it was down to the curry last night or the nerves today).

At midday we logged on, just in case the results were online early . . . they weren't. Kept checking, every five minutes or so until it got to 12.30p.m. Whilst all this was going on my daughter, who had broken up from school a day earlier than my son for half-term, had invited three friends round for lunch (two of them boys), and I was trying to bake bread and cook noodles and supply drinks . . . absolute chaos. I checked the clock and it had just gone 12.30. Clicked refresh on the online message board . . . shut my eyes and prayed . . . opened my eyes to find the message board looked exactly the same as it had done for the last half an hour. Spent ten minutes repeatedly clicking refresh and got the same thing every time – no results, bloody uni are so shite . . . ARRRGGGHHH!

Text the other girls who were waiting and they had already started ringing the uni trying to get hold of somebody, anybody who could clarify what was going on. I started ringing too; every single number I tried went straight to voicemail. How frustrating! Can't say we were surprised though. It's been like this all the way through with the bloody useless uni. They couldn't organise a piss-up in a brewery. They are more than useless. After spending an hour getting progressively more pissed off, the man in the know rang me (in reply to an irate voicemail message I had left) and informed us the results were now online. Panic! Couldn't thank him enough! Was trying to get back to the right Internet page, my bloody computer decided to freeze. Why does that always happen at THE most crucial moments? The results suddenly appeared . . . I got 68%! 68% is a 'B' . . . 2% off an 'A' (bugger) but a brilliant result (the highest in the group). Relief washed through me instantly, was one more hurdle that I had managed to get through. The entire group passed, that was the main thing. Sent the now-traditional results text to friends and family and immediately started getting congratulations messages back.

Sad as it is, I calculated my results average; am still aiming for a first, even though I said I wasn't! So far my results have been 74%, 60%, 69%, 74% and now 68% . . . add them up and divide by five and it gives 69% – 1% off the 70% I need to get my first! That means that with these final three essays, I need to average 75% to boost my overall average to 70%. Have got 75% once before in the first lot of submitted essays, although when averaged out between the three which were submitted the final mark was 74%. I need to try and pull out all the stops. My motivation to do that has returned and I am going to re-do two of the final three essays I have just completed and make sure they are the best I can possibly do. I am also going to book a tutorial with my personal tutor so I can get her input on how best to achieve this final goal. Am all excited again at the prospect of doing it! It's going to be hard work, but will be worth it . . .

Have two weeks till the summative OSCEs, then another two weeks to hand in these final essays and complete my final clinical assessment. Oh, and work full-time on delivery suite . . . so will have to spend every waking hour working hard.

Week Seventy

Wednesday

Have enjoyed a weekend at my mum's with the children in Norfolk, and a day in London yesterday. So no midwifery work done at all . . . Ooops! Coming down to earth with a bang now though. Have only ten days till summative OSCEs so need to revise, and still write the final essay (my tutor can see me for a tutorial on Monday, so five days to get the final one done). Also got off-duty for delivery suite for the next three weeks and it's all nights, so no chance at all of getting anything done . . . it completely buggers me up and I can only just function, let alone write essays and revise. Fan-bloody-tastic! Will also need to ask my little brother if he'd come and stay at mine the nights I'm working so the kids have someone here with them.

On a brighter note, one of the girls in my group has her interview at my Trust this morning. She popped in first thing to borrow my parking card, and I am waiting for her to return! Hope she does well, would be really lovely for us to all end up working together!

Friday

Still no revision done. Have managed to read all the research for my final essay, and start putting it together, so do feel as if I have achieved something! Also changed my shifts for delivery suite; am still doing nights, but have the weekend off prior to the OSCEs for what will be my only revision. Feel awful about it, I always prep really thoroughly for exams, and not being able to do that this time makes me feel even more nervous than I usually feel. Guess I could have made the effort in the evenings to revise, but am so knackered after looking after the kids all day that all I can do is climb into bed and sleep.

Son has been the usual handful this week . . . daily battles of will. Kept him occupied all morning scooping the insides out of three pumpkins we bought and he looked on the Internet for templates so we could make jack-o'-lanterns. They are all sitting on the kitchen side waiting for darkness to fall! We found an old CD of scary Halloween music, and have been listening to it whilst making a huge sticky mess! Off to visit family down south tomorrow.

Feel rather daunted by the fact I will be returning to delivery suite. I love it there, but often feel stupid and awkward. Only have twelve more deliveries to get, so hopefully I can relax and build up some much-needed confidence.

Week Seventy-one

Monday

Alarm went off at 6.30a.m. Was a real shock to the system getting up that early. It was dark and cold and all I wanted to do was stay in my nice warm bed. Managed to get myself up, make the packed lunches for the day and woke the children at 7a.m. We were washed and dressed and ready to leave the house at 7.30a.m. The plan was for daughter to stay on her own till school bus arrived across the road at 8 and for me to drive son to my brother's house for the day as sister-in-law was looking after him (teacher training day). Daughter decided she didn't want to be in the house on her own, and then got a text from sister-in-law saying could I take son to brother's work and meet there. Daughter ended up at father-in-law's for half an hour and I ended up in a traffic jam with son! Arghhhhhh!

Got to uni to find car park full. Parked under a tree in a muddy puddle. Made it into uni with minutes to spare. All the girls were there and we sat and had a coffee. By 9.15 we were starting to wonder where our lecturer was, and went to find her, only to find that she is on annual leave! Bloody uni! Typical. This was our last chance to get some support from the lecturers for our OSCEs, which are a week today away, and we were meant to have some practice stations set up so we could go through all the emergency stuff. The two other lecturers who should have been helping had not shown up either, so we all went out for a fag. On the way back through the car park we bumped into one of the missing lecturers who was still trying to park. She told us that there was no room booked for us that day and said we should all go home and revise. Now, I have a forty-mile round trip to uni, some of the girls travel even further than that, so we weren't best pleased by this. I ended up staying in uni for an hour, getting some books from the library and then seeing my personal tutor for some advice about my final trio of essays. I got some brilliant advice from her, and feel more confident about completing my essays (even though I have to change the focus of one of them completely). Disappointed with the general lack of support though; the OSCEs are our big exams, and for our only proper revision day to be fucked up like that just goes to prove yet again that if any of us manage to pass this course it won't be because of the support and guidance we have had from the university . . .

Got back to mine to find that two of the girls in my group were waiting outside and we had a revision session for the rest of the day. Sounds productive, but we only managed to cover pre-eclampsia and shoulder dystocia, but know them both inside out now, so feel a bit better. We spent the rest of the time helping one of them to rearrange her wedding, which was fun, and she had got herself into a right state about it, so am hoping we helped her feel better.

Feel more positive about revision now anyway. Am going to try and do some more tonight, and then have all day tomorrow before my first night shift. Hopefully I can crack on and get lots more done.

Tuesday

Had every intention of revising all day . . . didn't quite work out that way! Fellow student midwife who failed her exam had an interview at my Trust this morning, and she popped in with her hubby on the way home. She looked happy and confident and it sounded like the interview had gone well, and we spent an hour talking about it. When they left, I went online to check my emails, and two of the other girls in my group were chatting on MSN . . . that was it then for about two hours! Hee hee hee . . .

Had just started my revision (antepartum and postpartum haemorrhage in the community setting) and the phone rang. Fellow student midwife who had been interviewed this morning had got the call and been offered the job! That's three out of my group of five who will be working together. Half an hour later, the other girl in my group who was interviewed last week also got the call, and was also offered the job! All four of us together, fabulous!

Managed to get through the basics of APH (antepartum haemorrhage) and PPH (postpartum haemorrhage) along with the management from a midwives perspective before having to stop and collect son from school. Starting to feel nervous now. Have my first night shift on delivery suite tonight. Haven't been on delivery suite in my own Trust for six months, and I know as a senior student midwife they will be expecting a lot from me. Just hope I can remember everything and fingers crossed get a nice catch!

Wednesday

Got to delivery suite last night and the board looked quite full . . . made a cup of tea and waited for handover. Only one lady was labouring, the others were being transferred over to the postnatal ward. I wasn't allocated the labouring lady because another student (from an alternative Trust) piped up that as it was her last night, could she do it? She was told 'no' because there was a medical student in the room already! Ha ha ha . . .

I was allocated the care of a lady who was coming in. She was thirty-eight weeks pregnant with a history of abdominal pain and vomiting. She arrived about half an hour later and I was left to get on with it on my own (pretty daunting when it's been so long since being on delivery suite . . . hey ho). I took a history, did her obs and popped her onto a CTG. Everything was fine. Checked her urine which contained protein and ketones (which confirmed she was dehydrated) – informed the midwife in charge who advised to get docs in to review her. She had a vague history of SROM (spontaneous rupture of membranes) yesterday. Docs wanted me to do a speculum to check if liquor was leaking and to take bloods. Did speculum, no liquor, took HVS (high vaginal swab) and took bloods. Docs diagnosed a tummy bug and sent her home.

The ward rang with an induction lady (multip) who had just SROM'd and was requiring pain relief. I went to get her and was horrified when the midwife giving me handover also gave me a ten-page birth plan that 'must be adhered to'. This was going to be a disaster then; always was when women were trying to control every aspect of their labour. She looked in discomfort, but when I got her back to delivery suite and discussed pain relief she said she didn't want any. Again my mentor left me to it. Fetal heart was fine and I listened intermittently with a sonic aid. Her partner arrived soon after. He was very controlling and kept trying to get me to give her pain relief when she was saying she didn't want any . . . arrrgggghhh! She did request pain relief nearly two hours later and I went and checked with my mentor, asking if I could do a VE to check her progress first as it had been nearly four hours. She agreed and we went back into the room together. I did a VE and she was fully dilated, and immediately started pushing. Baby girl was born within twenty minutes . . . my twenty-ninth catch! She wanted a physiological third stage, and had no risk factors, so this was agreed. After twenty minutes she said she just wanted it over with and requested Syntometrine to help speed up the process. Her partner at this point started on about how it wasn't in the birth plan, and not to have the injection. We ignored him and let her get on and make the decision that was best for her, and she did have the injection. Placenta and membranes were delivered five minutes later! I popped the placenta into the receiver and scooped up a large clot and put it on the top. Then picked up the receiver and turned and put it on the trolley behind me . . . as I turned the clot slid off the top of the placenta and landed with a huge splatter on their birth plan – the ten-page birth plan that had to be adhered to (and wasn't at all). Was mortified . . . mentor thought it was hilarious and couldn't hide her laughter . . . gutted! Outside the room, she said she wished I'd aimed better and made it land on the husband's foot. Would have shown him!

Mentor went off for her break, and I did the baby check, gave vitamin K, completed all the computer bits, finished off the paperwork and transferred her back across to the ward and then went for my break. Got up at 6a.m. Had a cup of tea and some toast and then mentor said I could leave as no-one else was in labour and the morning shift would be coming on within the hour. Got home by 7a.m. and got kids to school and on school bus and was tucked up in bed by 8.30a.m. Bliss!

Back again tonight . . . different midwife in charge, so hoping now I have been eased back into things I will be able to prove myself a bit better tonight.

Thursday

Felt like a complete useless burden last night. All my confidence drained . . . was given a first time mum to care for. Epidural in situ, not working fantastically and needing Entonox; 4cm dilated 3 hours ago. I went in and introduced myself, felt like I didn't know what was going on. Popped a catheter in and did a VE. Now 6cm dilated, so progress slow but acceptable. Mentor came in and decided to start running Synto infusion as contractions were irregular and unco-ordinated. Just felt like I had no expertise on how to manage the situation; mentor asked me a few basic questions and I completely forgot everything I know, looked like a right lemon. Confidence on the floor. Trying to stop myself from bursting into tears and leaving and never returning . . . was pants.

Had a break at 3a.m. and woke up at 4a.m. feeling like I still needed to prove myself. Was time for another VE and I did that (after mentor) and she was fully dilated! Hooray! Due to epidural we allowed an hour for descent of the fetal head and at 5.50a.m. we started pushing. A huge baby girl was delivered at 6.30a.m. Mum coughed the head out, and vomited the body out . . . bless her. Completed the baby check and paperwork and handed her over to the morning staff. Got home in time to take son to before school club and then slept (badly) from 8.30a.m. till 2.30p.m. Feel drained; am dreading going back tonight at 9p.m. Can't begin to imagine what my mentor said about me to the rest of them last night and this morning – that I was shite probably. Why do I keep putting myself through this? Makes me wonder again whether I really want to do this after all.

To top things off, son has been in trouble at school twice this week. Why can't he behave and why can't I have a normal stress-free life?

Friday

Wow . . . Confidence back 100%! Feel on top of the world (apart from the fact I am knackered and sitting here with puffy eyes, waiting for man to come and put a new windscreen on my car, big crack . . . another £75 I hadn't budgeted for). Last night was amazing.

Board had a handful of women when the shift started. I was working with another midwife who I hadn't worked with before but everyone said she was really lovely, and she was – big relief! Took over the care of a woman in labour with her third baby who had been 7cm at 8p.m. She was using Entonox and had pethidine, which had taken the edge off the pain. Mentor was also midwife in charge, so she left me to it. My lady coped well for about forty-five minutes and then she lost it, requesting an epidural and verbalising the pain loudly! Between the contractions I got her consent to do a VE to assess her progress before siting an epidural; she agreed and I went to check this was OK with mentor, who also agreed. Returned to room and heard the fetal heart rate (FH) had dropped to about 80bpm . . . repositioned her but couldn't pick up FH again so pressed buzzer for mentor. Mentor came just as my lady gave a huge involuntary push . . . vertex was visible! My lady then started shouting at the top of her voice 'My minge ain't big enough ... my minge ain't big enough ... my minge ain't big enough'. Just managed to get delivery pack open and gloves on and baby's head was on the perineum! Another push and baby was delivered – all 10lb – huge baby! Checked perineum and it was intact, although she had a nasty labial tear which needed suturing. Mentor did that whilst I did baby check and gave vitamin K, then I sat at midwives' station and did paperwork to a chorus of 'my minge ain't big enough' courtesy of the other midwives who had heard my lady's shouts!

I had already been allocated the care of another woman who was making her way in with a history of her waters breaking and regular contractions. She arrived before I had completed the paperwork from my previous lady, but I left that on the side and took her to her room. She looked happy and comfortable and the midwife in charge apologised to me as we walked past (she knew I was desperate for deliveries) and this woman definitely did not look like she was in labour. Whilst talking to her and taking a history, she did stop regularly to breathe through contractions which were coming every two minutes. She then vomited a large amount. I managed to get her onto the bed to do an abdominal palpation, but before I had even listened into the FH she started screaming and pushing! I pressed the buzzer for my mentor, who had heard the screams and promptly arrived with the Syntometrine! Again, I just opened my delivery set and got my gloves on and the baby's head was on the perineum ... head restituted and I could see a hand up by the shoulder ... anterior shoulder began to deliver ... and baby was born. Tiny little thing, just over 5lb. Lady had second degree tear, due to compound presentation (hand getting in the way basically) that mentor sutured quickly. So I had delivered two babies within two hours ... bring it on!

The board was now looking horrendous. The on-call midwife had been called in and so far five babies had been delivered on our shift; two by me, one by another student and two by emergency section. All the rooms were full. There was also a high-risk lady on her way in with a history of drug abuse and domestic violence with a very unstable violent partner; police presence at all times had been advised. The police had been called and were on their way too. A grade four placenta praevia (the entire placenta covers the cervix blocking the baby's way out!) who had been on the ward had started contracting and she was being brought over; another lady from the ward had very high blood pressure so she was coming over, and a community midwife was on her way in an ambulance with a woman who had SROM'd with thick meconium and the fetal heart rate was below 80bpm (normal FH is 110-160bpm) . . .

The rest of the night was a blur. I wasn't allocated anyone myself to look after, instead I was flitting from room to room helping the midwives in any way possible. Was manic!

So, after getting home and sleeping for a few hours, phone going three times, and mobile buzzing away I am up and waiting for windscreen to be done. Have the whole weekend of revising to look forward to, OSCEs on Monday and then back to delivery suite for another three nights. With essays to finish and a formative and summative assessment to complete, I will be glad when this month is finished! Daughter is off out to the cinema with her friends this evening, and am just hoping son has had a good day at school (fingers crossed!).

Week Seventy-two

Monday

Feel absolutely gutted. Have terrible feeling that I have failed at least one of the OSCE stations. After spending the whole weekend revising with a friend from my group at her house, then she stayed at mine last night to revise some more, I couldn't have been any more prepared in the time we had. We were up till 1a.m. last night, and up again at 6a.m. this morning. Traffic on the way there was horrendous, *déjà vu* of last exam when exactly the same thing happening. . . busy motorway, our back route chock-a-block and having to speed excessively to get to uni, arriving twenty minutes late.

First station was written station . . . advice we would give to reduce the risk of cot death. Not revised it, but feel hopeful that I did enough to get through.

Second station was a demonstration station . . . shoulder dystocia, had revised it and felt quite confident when performing the manoeuvres. Third station was another demonstration station . . . explaining maternal serum screening. Hope I said the right things.

Fourth and final station was a VIVA, an oral station. PPH. Feel like I completely messed it up. Went through everything, but didn't once mention documentation, and really believe that they can't pass me on this because it's a key factor. Also discussed manual removal of the placenta which the midwife may have to do in an emergency situation, but don't think the way I said it demonstrated safe practice.

Now feel depressed and disappointed, that after all that hard work I may have failed something. I am on nights for the next two weeks. Have three essays to finish, a portfolio to complete and formative and summative assessments all to be finished within three weeks. I have four days off when the children are at school and will have to get it all done. The pressure is immense. Just can't help questioning whether it is all worth it. Really wish I could sit and cry, but the tears don't seem to want to come . . .

To top things off have just checked my off-duty allocations and have been given another week of nights, making four weeks in a row. Have sent a polite but firm email back saying I am not doing it. They can go jump as far as I'm concerned. The midwives don't have to do that so why should I? I am a single mum, and don't see my kids enough as it is doing this bloody course . . . If they don't like it – tough.

Tuesday

Got up feeling a little better. Kids off to school. Came back home with every intention of working on my essays all day . . . didn't quite go to plan!

Felt terrible for leaving uni yesterday without saying goodbye to one of the girls, so decided to give her a quick ring. We chatted about yesterday and went through how we thought we'd done. The postman shoved the usual pile of junk mail through the door and for some reason I picked it up whilst we were chatting and had a nose through. There was a large white envelope with the uni stamp on it – bloody hell, results. Still on the phone, opened envelope . . . 'Dear All, I have managed to get agreement that your results can come out promptly. Here are your feedback sheets from today's OSCEs. Please read the comments carefully. Your second attempt OSCEs will take place on (three weeks time) in the afternoon'. Don't have to be Sherlock Holmes to realise that I haven't passed them all then . . . Station one, reducing the risk of cot death . . . pass! Station two, shoulder dystocia . . . pass! Station three, primary postpartum haemorrhage, fail (knew that was coming). Station four, maternal serum screening . . . pass! Read them out over the phone as I checked each one. My hands were shaking. Emotionally, I was yo-yoing between relief and disappointment. At least I only have to re-sit one station. Sent the mandatory text to the other girls, all of whom replied asking how I knew my results . . . none of them had the post yet that morning.

Got off the phone and immediately rang my mum. She is going to have children for the weekend before the re-sit, so I can revise. Bless her. Phone rang as soon as I put it down and it was one of the girls (the one who had had to sit her written exam three times). She had failed three of the four stations and was distraught. Tried to encourage her as much as possible, but it was difficult. Got off the phone to her and it rang straightaway – again was one of the girls (the one I had revised with all weekend). She had failed the same one as me, and passed the others. We arranged the revision weekend at hers again for the re-sit. Got off the phone, it rang and the girl I had spoken to first thing had just got her letter. She had also failed the same one as us, but passed the others. Only one of the girls now left to get her results, but she was working a long day today and wouldn't be home to get her letter till this evening.

Knew deep down that I had failed the PPH station; should be

happy that I passed the others, but instead, I am dreading having to go through it all again. Anyway, start my nights tonight. Am doing tonight, tomorrow and Thursday . . . just hoping that my confidence continues to grow. Am working with a lovely midwife for this week. Although we have to do a formative clinical assessment by the end of the week, after only working three nights together, and then I have to do a summative assessment two weeks later, after not working with her at all after this week. God knows what she is going to think about it all. Have to have a chat with her tonight and see what she says. Fingers crossed she agrees to do it. Although I am well and truly buggered if she says no, because I work with a different mentor each week, so have no continuity. Hey ho.

Wednesday

Got to delivery suite last night to find the board completely empty! No women there at all! And, they had only had one elective Caesarean all day, so all the cleaning and tidying had been done. Sat and had a chat with my mentor about the assessments I needed to do with her, which she agreed to, and also discussed the skills I needed to practise. Made the most of the time by printing off loads of policy documents in regards to emergency situations, which hopefully will help when revising for the re-sit I have to do. Then we sat and watched a horror movie in the coffee room, frightening ourselves witless, and having to then go in pairs to the loo (down a dark and empty corridor at 2a.m.).

The phone rang and it was a first time mum who was contracting and not coping with the pain. I was allocated her care and she arrived within half an hour. I did a VE and she was already 7cm dilated, with bulging membranes. I looked after her for an hour and then was sent on my break. Got back a little while later and she was in the pool. Pain was getting more intense but her contractions were becoming irregular, so I did another VE and she was fully dilated . . . I also did an ARM (artificial rupture of membranes) to see if that would make her contractions more regular. By this time, the morning staff were coming on and although I would have stayed with this lady, it was a preceptorship midwife taking over, who was still being shadowed by an experienced midwife, so it wasn't really appropriate for me to stay too. My lady cried when I said I was going, but I promised her that I would pop and see her this evening before starting my night shift. Can't wait to go and meet her little baby!

Managed to sleep from 8.45a.m. till 2.45p.m. today, so not feeling too tired at the moment, although I am sure it will catch up with me in the early hours! Checked my emails quickly a moment ago; the advice we now have from one of the lecturers is that the same topics may come up in the OSCEs re-sit, although we had previously been told that they definitely wouldn't. Typical of that uni, they don't know their arse from their elbow. Will email all the lecturers and try and get some clarification on that . . . it hugely impacts what I need to revise.

Thursday

Devastated after last night's shift. Looking after a first time mum, did first VE at 2.30a.m. and found she was 6cms dilated. Thought she was heading towards second stage nicely due to involuntary pushing, so did another VE at 6a.m. – fully dilated. Got her pushing for an hour and presenting part was not visible, so mentor did another VE only to find she had an anterior lip. Pants. Was sure she was fully dilated. Completely lost my confidence and felt shite. I'd had her pushing on an anterior lip for an hour, so the risk of the lip of cervix being swollen and then acting as a barrier against the baby's descent was great. She did deliver vaginally about an hour later, but I was still gutted. Had worked right through the night, no break, and finished half an hour late, so didn't get to see kids this morning before they went off to school. Came home sad and tired.

Phone woke me up at 10a.m. then a delivery driver knocked on the door at 11a.m. even though I put a note on the door saying I am working nights and do not disturb . . . aaarrrggghhh! If he had knocked a second time he would have got an earful.

Hubby arrived to babysit for the night. Stormed in and immediately asked whether I had contacted the CSA, so he must have got his letter today. He grabbed all his stuff and walked out saying he would never look after the children for me again to cover my working hours. Fucking fabulous. Had to ring delivery suite and explain what had happened. Completely messes everything up because I was meant to do my formative assessment with my mentor tonight and she now has to judge my practice after working only two shifts together. Am not going to let it get to me. Have to rally my family round me and get on with completing the course, without having to rely on him for anything.

Friday

Woke up with a stinking headache probably caused by drinking three quarters of a bottle of white wine last night! Ha ha ha . . . Spent an hour chatting to fellow student midwife I had revised with, apparently the student midwife who had failed her exam twice and has now failed three OSCEs had a melt-down on delivery suite yesterday; hope she's OK, have sent her a text. Am now trying to stop myself from logging onto Facebook and make myself instead knuckle down and get these bloody essays finished.

11p.m.

Have had an awful evening. Son went to youth club . . . picked him up an hour and a half later to find that he had punched another little boy (the one who winds him up constantly at school). The little boy had a huge red mark under his eye, and his father was obviously livid (as I would be if it happened to my son). I apologised, and tried to calm the situation – my son wouldn't admit to doing it although two other people had seen it happen. Got him home and talked to him and he did eventually tell me the truth. These boys had been goading him all evening and he lost his temper. Didn't know what to do, so rang the parents of this other boy and spoke to his mother. She was angry but understanding, and thanked me for ringing and talking it through with her. Just feel like I am lurching from one crisis to another at the moment, don't know how much longer I can cope with it all.

Sunday

Got two lots of fantastic news! The first, on Friday, was an email from our cohort leader confirming that the OCSE re-sit is going to be the same scenario that we failed! That means no revising everything and anything like last time, but we can just concentrate on revising PPH (I have already printed the local Trust PPH policy so can use that for my revision). Means we really do have to bugger it up if we are going to fail again. What a huge relief!

Then yesterday I opened a letter from my solicitor that confirmed that my divorce will be finalised in two weeks' time! Still in a state of shock that it is happening this quickly, but not complaining. It's brilliant!!!

My family have got together to help cover all the childcare I need so I can carry on working and complete the course. Another huge relief. Now have two weeks before the final trio of essays goes in. Have completely finished one, after going back and making the changes my tutor suggested. The second one is in the process of being re-written, again with the changes my tutor suggested, and I am hoping that I can get that one finished tonight when the children go to bed. The third one is half-written, and I will need to get that one finished during the week. I am working Monday, Tuesday and Sunday nights, so will have Monday, Thursday and Friday to work on it whilst the kids are at school. The following week I am back on day shifts, so won't have that luxury, and then the essays are due in on the following Monday (my divorce day!).

Week Seventy-three

Wednesday

Has been another whirlwind few days. Hubby was told by CSA he had to pay more than what he thought he could pay and phoned me in a rage, demanding to come round and see *his* children ... Nightmare!

Work has been good. On nights again. Got to delivery suite Monday night and was given a lady who had just reached fully dilated! Fabulous! She was high-risk, and on a CTG with Synto running to augment her labour. Baby quickly became distressed and we had to rush her to theatre for an emergency section. Recovered her for a couple of hours after and then took over the care of another first time mum who was just getting into the pool for pain relief. She was 6cm dilated. On taking over I immediately saw she was not coping with the contractions and she was asking for further pain relief. I explained her options to her; basically she could only stay in the pool if she used Entonox, if she wanted anything stronger she would have to get out. I encouraged her to stay in the water through a few more contractions to see if it helped her relax, but prepped some Meptid for her if she needed it. She then completely got in her zone and started breathing through the contractions like an absolute star! Within an hour she said she was feeling the pressure to push, and we could see anal dilatation and that her bowels had been open, so we told her to listen to what her body was telling her to do and push if she really felt the urge was too much to breathe through. By this time it was gone 1a.m. I was knackered, dripping wet and was leaning over the pool scooping out poop with a sieve. Couldn't help but think to myself what a bizarre job I have! She progressed really well and after about half an hour's pushing, her baby's head was visible. We were using a mirror and torch to see, so we could tell her when to pant. Baby's head was delivered and it was the most surreal experience to look down into the water and see a little face looking up at me! Her bottom was close to the base of the pool so we flipped her into a kneeling position to give the baby's body space to be delivered, and she was . . . a beautiful little girl born in the water. Wonderful! Mum and her baby sat in the water for a few minutes, and then she got out to deliver her placenta. Was a perfect delivery and she was very proud of herself – quite rightly so.

A little while later another first time mum came in thinking she was in labour. She was huffing and puffing away, but her contractions were not palpable. She was asking for pain relief, so I did a VE expecting to then be sending her home because she wasn't in labour, but she was 6cm dilated! Got her some Meptid, started her on Entonox and by that time the morning girls came in to take over. Had a brilliant shift. Came home to sleep and managed to get five hours before getting up to do it all over again.

Got to delivery suite for my second night shift and was allocated the care of a young woman who had been in four times already thinking she was in established labour. She was very tired and very emotional. She would swing from politeness to absolute foul rudeness, and it was draining trying to care for her. This time her contractions were strong and she was asking for pain relief so I did a VE. She was 6cm dilated with bulging membranes, so I did an ARM. This didn't quite go to plan. I tried and tried to rupture her membranes, but just couldn't get them to pop. My mentor was getting shirty with me, and I gave up and let her have a go. She couldn't do it either! Had to get another amni-hook and she managed it straightaway, so must have been a dodgy one we were using first. She laboured well for about three hours and then started getting strong urges to push, although they were intermittent. I did a VE and she had an anterior lip, which I was able to gently push over the baby's head. She then started pushing like a trooper and the baby was born within an hour. By 4.30a.m. she had showered and settled back for a rest and I was sent for my break. I asked them to wake me, as I was knackered and worried that I would not wake myself after an hour. I woke up myself a little while later and it was 6.45a.m. They had let me sleep for over two hours. Got up and had a cuppa, but nothing was happening on the ward so I was sent home!

Got home feeling wide awake after my sleep. Chatted to fellow student midwife who had three attempts at first exam and has just failed three of the four OSCEs. She saw tutor yesterday and has basically been told that she doesn't have enough time to complete the work she needs to in order to pass. In fact, she said tutor had questioned why she was even going to bother trying! Great support yet again from uni. Tried to encourage her to get her head down and get through these last few weeks, but she didn't sound convinced. Also chatted to one of the other girls in my group, who has been going through the same highs and lows that I have . . . questioning her abilities and knowledge and losing confidence, getting it back and losing it again . . . Why are we doing this?!

Worked on essay till 1p.m. and realised that I need to sleep because I couldn't type a single word without make a typo! So took myself up to bed with the intention of sleeping for an hour. Woke up over two hours later, cutting short a wonderful dream where I had just started flirting with a hunky policeman! Solicitor rang, and said she would send me the papers to have my name changed, and she clarified that I won't actually be divorced in two weeks' time, but once it has gone to court I can apply for the final bit which takes a further six weeks. Bummer . . . had got myself excited about that, but at least I can change my name sooner rather than later! And my maiden name will appear on my midwifery degree too!

Kids have just gone to visit their dad for an hour, he has moved into the flat over the local pub (fabulous place to have children visit). Never mind. Am knackered, and just need more sleep. Have arranged to work in a gynae clinic for the morning tomorrow, so won't be able to have a lay-in either. But at least that's another bit of my portfolio which I can complete and not have to worry about.

Thursday

It's 10.30 at night. I have worked on my essay all day and have now had half a bottle of wine . . . can feel the room spinning, and finding it really hard to type. Best go to bed methinks!

Week Seventy-four

Monday

Worked last night. Was allocated the care of a woman expecting her second baby who wanted a vaginal birth after Caesarean (VBAC). My mentor let me get on with it and I popped her into her room when she arrived, did an initial assessment and hooked her up to the CTG because of previous section and history of SROM. CTG was good for all of fifteen minutes and then I observed some variable decelerations, so called my mentor in. That's when it all went tits-up. My mentor completely took over, doing all the VEs and basically I had nothing to do. Woman wasn't coping well, and was only 2cms dilated, and eventually ended up having an epidural.

In the meantime, my old mentor had been allocated the care of another woman expecting her second baby who was on her way in with a history of SROM. The old mentor (who I love to bits) came and grabbed me (knowing I have five shifts left to get five catches) and shoved me in the room with this lady when she arrived. She was very obviously fully dilated (anal dilatation and strong urges to push). All I managed to do was to introduce myself and get some gloves on and the baby was born . . . beautiful delivery. On checking the vagina and perineum afterwards I found a small first-degree tear. Usually they wouldn't be sutured, but this one was bleeding. We left the room to check the placenta and give Mum and Dad some time with their new daughter. I asked my mentor if I could do the suturing, and she agreed! I was so nervous . . . hands shaking . . . feeling sick. I got back into the room and prepped my trolley. Put lady in lithotomy. Drew up local anaesthetic. Completely crapped myself! Managed to get local anaesthetic in OK and sutured! With the help of my mentor whispering words of wisdom over my shoulder . . . I did it! I did it! I did it!

Wednesday

Yesterday's shift was OK. Didn't get any catches, but did have my final summative assessment. Bit of a drama around that one . . . here goes! Got to the hospital and parked as usual. Noticed that my community mentor's car was there. Thought it was a bit weird, as was only 7a.m. and my assessment not due till 10a.m. Walked up to delivery suite to find the place bursting at the seams. Everyone looked exhausted, and my poor community mentor looked awful. She had been there since midnight (after having worked a full day in the community yesterday), the board was full, and everyone was running around like headless chickens. The other mentor who was doing my assessment was meant to be on an early, but had been called at 5a.m. to come and start earlier.

Had handover. Community mentor said she would come back at 10a.m. for my assessment. I assured her that she needn't feel like she had to, and that I could sort something else out, but she was adamant, bless her, that she would be there. My delivery suite mentor said she probably wouldn't be able to leave delivery suite for the assessment but she would be more than happy to sign off all my paperwork afterwards and pop out and have a word with my tutor.

Took over the care of a woman in labour with her fourth baby who was 9cm dilated. My delivery suite mentor left me to it (scary!) and I went in to do what I had to do. She was starting to feel the urge to push, although there were no external signs of full dilatation. She couldn't stop herself from pushing, so I did a VE to assess her cervix. She had an anterior lip which I pushed over the baby's head. The FH dropped to 40bpm, so I pulled the emergency bell whilst changing her position to left lateral and it quickly recovered. The midwife in charge was in the room within seconds, and with the next contraction the FH dropped again, so I put her onto a CTG to monitor what was happening. The FH then stabilised and she carried on pushing. Her contractions seemed to be going off the boil, and after half an hour of pushing the head wasn't visible so I went to talk to my mentor. I asked her to do a VE to check that the anterior lip was gone, which she found it had. The lady's contractions had really slowed down now, so my mentor suggested popping in IV access and getting some fluids in to rehydrate her. We did this, and the doc came to review the CTG. It was planned to give her a little Syntocinon to get the contractions established again.

There was a knock at the door. It was 10a.m. already and my community mentor was there. My delivery suite mentor said it was OK for me to go to my assessment and she would carry on with my lady's care and call me if the delivery was imminent. So, grabbed a quick cup of tea and headed for my assessment. My uni tutor was also there and ready. Passed everything at level four (independent practice) and all the paperwork was signed! Yippee! My tutor said she wanted a quick word with my delivery suite mentor, so I returned to my lady's room . . . chaos! Doc and anaesthetist were there getting consent from her for an emergency Caesarean. Baby had become distressed and needed to come out quickly . . .

Mentor gave me the theatre paperwork to complete and went to send bloods off; I told her tutor was outside wanting a quick word. Was in theatre within a few minutes, and baby boy was born . . . all was OK. We were back in the recovery bay within the hour and I recovered her. Finally got a break at about 2.30, and mentor said tutor had gone for a coffee and never returned! Fabulous! She said she would still sign off all my paperwork, but we never got a chance that shift as things were still so busy.

Got to work the following day, praying it wasn't going to be quite as busy . . . ha ha ha, wishful thinking! Was getting changed into my scrubs and a student midwife who had been on the night shift was in there having a quick wee. She asked me if I still needed deliveries . . . yes, yes, yes! She said her woman was fully dilated and pushing, but she had to go home, did I want to take over? Well, got into my scrubs in seconds and went straight into the room. She was a first time mum and had been pushing for a couple of minutes . . . plenty of time then! Introduced myself, and calmed her down, and talked through what she was going to feel, what was going to happen, and what I would be saying to her to stop the head from being delivered too quickly.

She gave one almighty push and the head was visible! Got my delivery pack open, got my gloves on, and midwife who had been there with the other student went and got me some Syntometrine. A couple of pushes later and head was crowning. Baby boy was born within two minutes of me going into the room! Catch number thirty-seven! She had an intact perineum too . . . good for her! Got all her paperwork done, and was asked to go into theatre to do the elective section for that day. Did all this lady's theatre paperwork and escorted her to theatre. Anaesthetist had four attempts of siting IV access and failed . . . got another anaesthetist in, and she managed it after another couple of attempts. Spinal went in easily and I was asked to catheterise her in the left lateral. Could I do this? No I bloody couldn't. Consultant had to. Theatre staff were being really shirty because it had taken so long to get IV access and spinal in . . . like it was my fault! They finally started the section, but lady was complaining of a lot of pain, so the decision was made to give her a GA (general anaesthetic). Baby eventually delivered and again I did all the post-op care. Knackered, hungry and thirsty . . . I got home and went to bed when the kids did at 8p.m.

Thursday

Was a good day. Worked with a lovely midwife. Had a mum who was dilating slowly, labouring with her second baby. She had a Synto drip and was coping well with Entonox. CTG showed variable decelerations and we got doc in to review. Synto was switched off and we started to use more fluids to rehydrate her. She was very frightened, and her partner explained she hadn't had a very good experience the first time round, but she was doing well. Did a VE at 9a.m. and she was 5-6cm dilated. She got urges to push at about 10.30 and I did another VE; she had an anterior lip, which I pushed over the baby's head. She was quite a large lady, and obviously had quite a large baby on board, so my mentor and I had discussed the possibility of shoulder dystocia and PPH. She pushed well, and the presenting part immediately became visible. Head delivered very slowly . . . my mentor and I looked at each other both thinking 'fuck', shoulder dystocia, but head delivered with a trickle of fresh blood . . . baby restituted and blood continued. Head was deep purple/blue . . . body delivered with more blood. Baby didn't attempt to breathe . . . stimulated with towel and clamped and cut cord. Gave Syntometrine as bleeding continued. Rubbed up a contraction. Baby now breathing. Bleeding had stopped . . . Huge sigh of relief! At this point delivery suite manager popped her head around the door; she wanted us to take our other lady to theatre for her elective LSCS (breech presentation) . . . like we were able to! Madness. Placenta delivered easily and my mentor left me and went to get the other lady into theatre. I did the vitamin K, baby check, labelling and paperwork. Got tea and toast, booked a bed on the ward; she needed a few sutures, so couldn't get her to the shower straightaway.

Once mentor had caught baby in theatre, we swapped. I did post-op care and she went in to suture. I did all the computer bits and by that time, the afternoon shift were coming on duty, thank the Lord! We had a quick cup of tea, and then transferred first lady to the ward. She was very sweet, kept saying how she couldn't have done it without us, and how much she appreciated us helping her! Was lovely to get some praise! And it had been an honour caring for her. Got back to delivery suite and gave section lady a wash and then transferred her to the ward too. It was now half an hour after we were meant to finish and I still needed to get proper delivery suite midwife to sign my portfolio. She was in a room with a lady and a different student. Have really developed a good relationship with this midwife. She had scared the living daylights out of me when I first started, but I tried to put those thoughts behind me, and have made the effort to get along with her – she is lovely. Was still nervous about asking her if she had time to sign my portfolio, but didn't have a choice, because it goes in on Monday. So I knocked on the door and waited. She came out and I asked her if she had time to sign it. She said she did and came straightaway! I had labelled all the pages that needed signatures and she whipped through them all and wrote a wonderful comment at the end. Whilst she was doing this, the delivery suite manager was hovering behind us waiting to speak to her and they both said how well I had coped over the last few shifts and what a fantastic midwife I was going to be! Was wonderful to hear; I need to be more confident in my own abilities, and I always worry how other people view me, so was a real confidence boost!

Got home an hour late. Collapsed in a heap on the sofa. Daughter made me a nice cup of tea. A little while later I put dinner in the oven, and then forgot about it so it burned! Managed to make something else, have a bath and then we all fell into bed (8p.m. again!).

Friday

Have printed off my final three essays. Have packed my bag for the revision weekend. Roll on next week when the assessments will all be over!

Week Seventy-five

Monday

It's portfolio submission day! Have read and re-read my essays and have them all ready to hand in. Have scrutinised every single page of my two portfolio folders to make sure that every page is signed and dated as it is meant to be. My current overall percentage is 69%, although I am fighting to get my exam grade of 60% increased to 61% because it was 60.666 and all the other girls had their marks rounded up and mine was rounded down. If they do this, my overall grade will be 69.2% and I may still be able to get a first if these last three essays get 74% or 75%.

Revision was good . . . got lots done, and drank lots of wine too!

Am off to uni in a mo to get these essays and portfolio submitted. Will be such a relief!

8p.m.

Fellow student midwife who I had revised with for the weekend came to mine and we made our way to uni. Handed my portfolio and essays in! Was waiting for the relief to sweep over me, but it never came. Now worried about what mark I will get and whether it's enough for a first! Anyway, got to uni expecting student midwife who had three attempts at exam to be there having a one-to-one with our cohort leader. She had failed three out of the four OSCEs and the rest of us decided not to go for the full revision session, because there was no need to go over the other two topics as we had passed. Walked into classroom and three-attempts-at-exam student midwife wasn't there. Lecturer was livid, but chatted to us, and we revised PPH together. None of us could believe that the other student midwife had not done the revision session. Lecturer said her car had broken down; I got a text saying her car was having an MOT. Lecturer basically told us this was our last and final attempt at passing, and that we would not complete the course if we don't pass the re-sit OSCEs on Wednesday. No pressure then . . .

Tuesday

Revision weekend student midwife arrived at mine at 9.30a.m. followed by one of the other student midwives in my group. We spent till 3p.m. revising, reading, revising, discussing, revising. Our brains were quite numb when we stopped! Got son from school and revision weekend student midwife was staying the night, so we could carry on revising when kids went to sleep. Indian takeaway for tea . . . yummy! Kids in bed, wine open and flowing freely we got back to work. Stopped at 11p.m. and watched *I'm a Celebrity... Get Me Out of Here* (recorded earlier in the evening on Sky plus!) and headed to bed. Son woke me up at 2.30a.m. I remember jumping and yelling PPH! Frightening the life out of student midwife who was sharing my bed . . . ha ha ha . . .

Wednesday – make or break day

Waves of nausea, panic and constipation keep hitting me! This is it. Fifteen minutes this afternoon is going to decide my fate. Am I ever going to be a midwife? Doesn't feel like it at the moment. Managed to make packed lunches for the kids. Daughter left to catch her school bus, got son to school with one minute to spare to find that it was non-school uniform day (he was in his uniform) so we came home and he changed. See, this is what this bloody course does to you . . . can't even organise my kids properly!

Sat and revised, chain-smoked and drank at least another ten cups of tea waiting for the other girls to arrive. We were all ready by 11a.m. and we were off. Bloody miracle but the usually horrendous road from hell that we have to drive down to get to uni was accident-free and we made it into the city by 11.30. Stopped to buy teabags and lots of doughnuts, cookies and cakes and headed to uni. Tea had filled our bladders to their capacity but our cohort leader ambushed us en route to the loo and said she needed to speak to us urgently . . . panic! She gave us the timetable for that afternoon's OSCEs and it had been rearranged (as we had previously requested) so all the stations were running simultaneously. This meant that instead of me waiting two and a half hours in exam conditions for my turn, I was only waiting an hour and five minutes (I was last). Fabulous! She also said we all needed to meet at the end and we mustn't disappear home as and when we finished . . . Wonder what that's about?

Had time to pee, another cup of tea and a fag . . . then we were off. One by one we were called into the dreaded room . . . first out, happy face . . . second out, burst into tears, had run out of time . . . third out, very quiet . . . fourth out, tears but smiling . . . my turn. Fuck. Remember going in, sitting down. Lecturers both had smiles, and were being kind. Put my watch in front of me and read scenario. Exactly the same as before, relief! Started talking, blurted out everything I could remember, trying to get it into order, was playing with my pen. Popped the lid off and it flew through the air, hitting the wall. Completely lost it at that point and apologised for sending things flying around the room! Lecturers were both laughing hysterically . . . great! Got back into my zone and carried on, said everything I needed to, had two minutes left; lecturer asked me what the definition of a PPH was, told her, she asked me if there was anything else I would do afterwards . . . think think think . . . what had I missed . . . repeated things I had said already . . . aaarrrggghhh! Looked up and she was miming writing something . . . documentation! I had said that, but said it again. She carried on miming the same thing . . . fluid balance chart. I had said that too, but said it again . . . The miming continued. And then it came to me. Incident report form . . . debrief with Supervisor of Midwives, debrief student midwife. It all came spilling out and I just finished as she pressed stop on the tape recorder. Shakily got up and walked out of the room. The other girls were waiting and we went for another cup of tea and another fag.

We all trudged cold and exhausted back into the classroom. Our cohort leader was in the exam room with another lecturer and some people we didn't recognise and they were all deep in conversation. We waited, and waited, and waited . . . they didn't come out. After forty-five minutes, we all trudged back outside into the cold to have yet another fag. Back into classroom, waiting, waiting, waiting . . . After another thirty minutes she came in. She was at a loss for words. She basically told us that she wasn't in a position to tell us our results straightaway, and that we would hear by the middle of next week. Our minds all went into overdrive. If we had all passed we would have been told today, surely? Was it that one or more of us have failed? Was it that if one person had failed, they didn't want to give us the news in front of the others? Was it that the markers can't agree? Was it because if someone has failed it needs to be moderated before the final decision can be made and we get kicked off the course, with three weeks to go? Three weeks to go for God's sake . . . Am questioning now whether I said the right things. Did I get my drug doses mixed up? Did I forget something really obvious? But just can't remember, it really is a blur.

Again, that expected wave of relief never came. We sat in the car silently driving home. No-one making the effort to speak; everyone crapping it in case today has sealed our fate never to become fully-fledged midwives. Want to cry. Want to scream. Want to shout. Want to quit. Want to control it somehow but it's too late. Have to sit tight and wait . . .

Thursday

Woken up by alarm clock at 6a.m. Dark, cold, and could hear the rain hitting the window. Did not want to get up, wanted to curl up into a ball and never move again, but needless to say I made myself. Went through the usual motions of making packed lunches, getting out the kids' school uniforms, getting their school bags ready, filling the dog's water bowl, putting newspaper down just in case . . . finally had a cup of tea.

Got to delivery suite ready for the 7.30a.m. start. Three women on the board. One postnatal, one in early labour and one with abdo pain but only thirty-four weeks pregnant. I got the abdo pain woman, who was in sooo much pain she couldn't go home, but was actually fast asleep in bed. Good. Time for another cup of tea! Yippee! Finally got too bored by 9.30a.m. and went and woke her up with some breakfast. Popped her on the CTG and all was well. As soon as I mentioned home, she started getting the pains again, and doc reviewed. We transferred her to the ward after giving her a couple of paracetamol.

Next I was allocated the care of a multip who had phoned in with regular contractions. Got room ready and waited for her to arrive. Waited, waited, waited . . . another two cups of tea later she rolled through the doors looking quite comfy, thank you very much. Did an initial assessment and popped her onto a CTG (previous section was the risk factor) and we sat and chatted. She was contracting regularly and looked like she was in labour but her care was allocated to another student midwife for the afternoon and I went off for my lunch.

Sat around for another hour with not a lot to do. Thirty minutes before I was due to go home, another lady was admitted and I did the initial assessment. This lass must have only been twenty and her partner was in his fifties . . . (unlikely couple!). Got home by 4p.m. Foul mood, tetchy, moody and miserable. Bloody uni for putting us through this shit. Am sure they take some ritualistic pleasure over torturing us all like this. Checked post, just in case, nothing. Checked answerphone, just in case – nothing. Checked email, just in case – nothing. Have a headache, feel awful and just want to sit and cry. It wouldn't be so bad if we knew when to expect the results, but we don't even know that. Got some text messages from the other girls. They all feel exactly the same. Think this must be the biggest low of the course so far.

Friday

Have been waiting for the postman all morning. He brought one letter, stamped with the uni logo. Shaking uncontrollably I managed (God knows how) to open the letter. It's not what I was hoping for, but good news all the same. My exam mark has been amended from 60% to 61%, and they have apologised for getting it wrong. That means I have to achieve a minimum average mark of 71% for this final trio of essays to get my first, which takes the pressure off a little. Still feeling sick . . . am on a late this evening, and an early tomorrow. Only need two more catches, but my heart really isn't in it at the moment- Want it all to be over.

11.30p.m.

Work was fab. Took over the care of a multip who had a section last time for breech, so had never laboured. She was just starting second stage and all I had to do was encourage her and talk her through it. She was pushing really well, but getting to the crucial point and backing away from the pain. We tried her in all sorts of positions, and even started fluids as her contractions became irregular, but after two hours the presenting part still slipped back between her contractions. My mentor suggested I do a VE to assess her perineum for an episiotomy, so I did. It was thick and not very stretchy so we made the decision (with her consent) to do an episiotomy. I injected the perineum with local anaesthetic, and with the next contraction did the episiotomy ... Didn't have time to be scared, and my mentor was right there talking me through it. Her baby girl was born and I had got catch thirty-nine! Was shaking whilst writing up the notes, had not expected to do an episiotomy, and felt quite sick afterwards.

Saturday

Will I get my number forty? The same question kept running through my head on the drive into work this morning. I got to delivery suite and was allocated the care of a first time mum who was 8cm dilated at 5a.m. meaning she should be heading into second stage very soon. She was labouring in the pool, and my mentor and I went and took handover. She was involuntarily pushing, and I explained to her that I needed to do a VE to ensure her cervix was completely gone. She stayed in the pool whilst I did this. She was fully dilated with bulging membranes, which ruptured as I was examining. Meconium stained liquor could be seen, so we had to move her out of the pool and pop her onto a CTG machine, just so the baby could be monitored continually.

She pushed for about an hour, and the presenting part was advancing nicely. My mentor was leaving me to it, popping in and out of the room. The presenting part did not slide back after a particularly fantastic push and I opened my delivery set, drew up my Syntometrine and buzzed for my mentor. She came through the door just as I delivered a big baby boy . . . the paed was right behind her (she had been called because of the meconium), but the baby was fine and paed wasn't needed. I had done it! Delivered baby number forty! I couldn't stop smiling, I danced my trolley out of the room and down the corridor and mentor had drawn a big number forty next to my woman's name on the board. Was an amazing feeling!

The rest of the shift was a bit of a blur. Mentor said I had done number forty so was now a proper midwife and gave me two women to assess who were possibly in labour. The first one arrived and asked me to examine her to see what was happening; she was 1cm dilated. I gave her the latent phase of labour spiel and sent her home. The second lady was the same, although I did a speculum because she was a possible SROM. Her cervix was not visible, and again I sent her home with the same advice.

Week Seventy-six

Tuesday

Should have been in uni yesterday, but son woke me up at 2a.m. and then vomited repeatedly right through the night. Needless to say he didn't go to school, and I didn't go to uni. He spent the day in bed, or on the sofa. I put the Christmas decorations up on the outside of the house, and we cuddled up and watched *Miracle on 34th Street* on the TV. He didn't eat anything all day, and although he was back to his usual self this morning, I phoned in sick and have kept him home. He is much better, although he still hasn't eaten anything.

I got a letter from my Trust about the planned change to working hours. Looks like I will be working long days when I start after Christmas . . . 7.30a.m. till 8p.m. Have requested that I don't do consecutive shifts, because the days I work I won't see the children, so it's not fair on them.

Still no news about OSCEs. Am fed up with it all now. Am glad I didn't make the effort to go to uni on Monday. The morning lecture ended up being an hour, and the girls hung around till 1p.m. waiting for the afternoon lecture only to get a message that it was cancelled. I would have been livid! Typical of that bloody uni though. Should know by now not to expect anything to be straightforward. Still have essay results to wait for too. Am back at work tomorrow for a late shift, and then an early on Saturday. I then have two days and two nights the week after, and my student days will be over. Oh my God . . . still can't quite believe it. Six shifts left as a student and then I will be a proper midwife, expected to do it all on my own. Cripes, that's scary . . .

Wednesday

Am completely disillusioned with everything. Still no news about OSCEs; was sure a letter would come today but it hasn't. Got so mad with all this waiting I rang the cohort leader. Thankfully for her she wasn't there . . . don't think I would have been able to control myself. Rang my personal tutor, she wasn't there. Rang another lecturer, she wasn't there. Rang the lady from the exam board, she wasn't there. Bloody university. Rang reception (who were there) and they put me through to another lecturer who could only say that the next exam board meeting was next week! I can't live another week with this pressure.

Rang one of the other girls, and we decided we would email the cohort leader, explaining how we felt (as if they didn't already know), so we did. She emailed us straight back (bloody miracle) but could only say she needed to check with exam board before posting our results online . . . lady from exam board off sick at the mo, so we are still in the dark about exactly when (and if) our results will be released.

Am working a late today. Have had a bath and washed my hair, and forced myself to eat lunch . . . feel sick and shaky . . . just want this whole nightmare to be over. Want to scream and shout and cry and get it all out of my system. Trying to hold things together, but don't think I can for another week.

The new eighteen-month programme is being planned at the moment and they want two from my group to go to a meeting (150 miles away) to give our opinions on the course we are doing. One of the girls who was going to go now has flu, and has asked me to go instead. I don't mind going, but I am not going to hold back on how crap the whole course has been from start to finish, and how disorganised and useless the uni and lecturers have all been. Hopefully the girls doing it next time won't have to put up with all this shit.

Just got back from the late shift. All went to pot really . . . took over the care of a first time mum who was fully dilated when I examined her. She had an epidural, so we would normally wait for an hour to allow descent of the fetal head, but her CTG was becoming abnormal. We had it reviewed by the doctor, and started second stage immediately. Within ten minutes the decelerations became late decelerations, and deep (down to 60bpm) and were slow to recover. We called the doc back and he examined and said fetal head was still in the transverse, and that he wanted to do an instrumental in theatre. So it was a mad dash to get her ready . . . We had a right to-do trying to get her into the lithotomy in theatre; the theatre staff didn't seem to know how to use the stirrups, and the epidural wasn't effective enough, so she ended up having a general anaesthetic (GA). It was a difficult instrumental and the baby came out floppy. Paeds were already there, and I took the baby to Resuscitaire where paed started resus. This paed was fab . . . he gave some inflation breaths which were very effective and within a couple of minutes baby was pink and crying.

My mentor had never recovered a GA patient before so I took over and did what was needed. Woman did give me a scare by remaining tachycardic (abnormally rapid heart beat, 150bpm) for quite some time, but we called the anaesthetist in and dealt with it. Delivery suite had calmed down and I managed to sit and have something to eat (a rarity for a midwife on duty!). I was then allocated the care of a twenty-five weeker who was coming in with abdo and back pain. I got the room ready and did the initial assessment. Things weren't quite as straightforward as I had thought. She was an ex-cocaine addict on methadone, with an alcohol problem. I got the docs into review, and they discharged her home after a couple of hours after giving her the all-clear.

Finished my shift feeling quite proud of myself. Had enjoyed the shift even though we had ended up in theatre. Give it a couple of weeks and I will be doing it all on my own.

Thursday

Alarm clock woke me up at 5a.m. Was out the door by 6a.m. and driving through the ice and darkness to fellow student midwife's house so we could make the journey together to uni for this meeting. Took me forty-five minutes to get to hers, and took us another hour and a half to get to the main uni campus, but got there on time.

We were briefed on the support aspects the lecturers thought the panel would quiz us on. Obviously they wanted us to sing their praises . . . didn't quite turn out that way once we were in front of the panel though! Surprise, surprise!! We spoke truthfully about the pressures of the course, the crap support we have had, the fact that we never quite know when we will get results, and it went on from there. They looked appalled at our experiences . . . rightly so. The lecturers have no idea what a shite time we have all had, they are too worried about their own egos and little power trips to seem to notice. We were done by 11a.m. and instead of going back and making small talk with the 'we love ourselves' lecturers, we scarpered and went for lunch!

Two of the girls in my group had their final assessments today. The first one passed with flying colours. The second one failed. She sent a brief text and I tried to ring her but there was no reply. I got another text an hour later saying she was waiting for them to make a decision about what was going to happen next, but apparently the lecturer had told her that it wasn't hopeful. We have a matter of weeks left on this course, and everyone knew she had been struggling since failing the exam twice in the first six months. It just seems so unfair to have kept her on the course this long, for her to be discontinued with a couple of weeks left. She is meant to be submitting her portfolio on Monday, which isn't completed yet, but she has been told not to return to practice, and to wait for the exam board to make its decision. I think deep down we all knew this was going to happen, and I think she did too, but the way it has been handled is yet another example of how crap this university is.

We also found out today that we will not know the results of our OSCEs until after the exam board meeting next Tuesday. So that means another week of torture, not knowing whether we will qualify or not . . . it really is the pits. Our whole futures rest on this, and they know the results, but can't tell us (or won't tell us, more like).

Saturday

Did all my Christmas shopping yesterday and then met fellow student midwife who has failed her summative assessment. She seemed to be coping with it all very well, and still in denial that she was not going to finish. She is applying for nursing jobs, and I encouraged her to do that. Deep down I think she knows she won't be a midwife, but can't accept it yet . . . it's dreadful.

I worked an early today; the professional development midwife was there and I was allocated to work with her. She told me that the plan for when I start will be an induction week, two weeks delivery, two weeks postnatal ward, two weeks day assessment unit, and two weeks community, then I can decide where I need to consolidate my skills the most and that can be arranged. We were allocated the care of two ladies who were on their way to the unit. The first was twenty-three weeks gestation with abdo pain; she looked awful when she arrived and I did an assessment, and bleeped the doctors to review her. My second lady hadn't arrived, but one of the other midwives had a para three who'd SROM'd and was showing anal dilatation. She grabbed me and hauled me into the room and I delivered the baby within five minutes! After checking the placenta, my mentor pulled me back out

271

and I carried on with my original lady. Got catch forty-one though, so that was good!

My original lady was being transferred to the ward and being put into isolation, so mentor sorted that whilst I did the assessment on the second lady. She had SROM'd thirty-eight hours previously and was coming in for induction of labour. Everything was normal and I popped her onto the CTG. Immediately I could see some decelerations, so I called senior midwife in to have a look. She asked me to do a VE and the lady was 3cm dilated. She called consultant in, and he was happy for Synto infusion to commence. So I got that ready and then I tried to site a cannula . . . I got it into the vein, but it wouldn't go in completely, so mentor did it for me. Am glad I tried though, was easy enough and it has helped to build my confidence doing it. It was only the second one I have ever attempted.

We got Synto started and I carried on caring for her. She decided she wanted an epidural so I arranged that and helped anaesthetist whilst she sited it. By this time the afternoon girls were taking over, so I handed over and went for lunch. Afterwards I took over again whilst new midwife had a break. There were now some deep decelerations which were late, so I called senior midwife in to look. She again called doc and it was decided that another VE was necessary (one was due in fifteen minutes anyway). She was fully dilated! Baby was direct OP but she was fully dilated! I explained to her that usually we would wait an hour for baby to descend, and then we would start her pushing. So if the baby behaved, that's what the plan would be. My shift finished, I had over my forty catches, I needed some mummy time myself, so I said my goodbyes and wished them luck. Will ring delivery suite shortly to see how she got on!

Whilst all that had been happening, I was talking to mentor. Just happened to mention about fellow student midwife who was possibly being discontinued and I went on to explain about the OSCE results being delayed and how worried we all were that it was us that had failed. Mentor just said 'You've got nothing to worry about, believe me . . .' and gave me a smile and a little wink. Maybe she knows somehow about what's going on but can't tell me officially. This has sort of put my mind at rest, but at the same time it hasn't. Anyhow, I have two days off now. Am spending tomorrow with my kids and then heading into town on Monday to sort out my change of name with the bank and building society. Still need to inform the DVLA and child tax and child benefit people too . . . what a fun day that's going to be!

Week Seventy-seven

Tuesday

OK, are you ready for the latest on the OSCE results? Well, it's complete and utter C. R. A. P. crap crap crap . . . One of the girls phoned me last night, she had seen one of the lecturers at the hospital yesterday whilst she was working. The lecturer had gone over to speak to her and she took the opportunity (yet again) to try and get confirmation of when our results are going to be given to us. The lecturer confirmed that the exam board meeting would be today, but she seemed surprised that we were all under the impression that the results would then be released straightaway. She said that the normal way of doing things is for the meeting to be held on a Tuesday and then the results would be made available to students on the Friday. Friday! Bloody hell, what are they trying to do to us? That will mean that we won't know whether we have passed or not until two days before the course finishes.

I can't take much more of this. They are continually moving the goalposts, and it's not fair. Should have expected this I suppose, based on their track record. The next thing will be that we won't know till after Christmas. If that happens I will go and see the Dean of the University myself, and camp on his doorstep till he sorts out this whole mess . . .

Just got a text from one of the girls and she has got her fortieth delivery with a physiological third stage! So two of us have now reached the magic number of forty, the others aren't far behind.

Yesterday I saw fellow student midwife who failed her summative; she popped over with her dog and we went for a walk over the fields together. It was really difficult. She should have gone for an interview in the Trust where she is training that morning. She had failed the first interview, but they were prepared to give her a second go . . . She didn't turn up; didn't ring them; email them or anything to let them know she wasn't going. She kept saying that there was no way the uni would discontinue her now because she was so close to the end, and that she had a job lined up in the Trust I work in, so she wasn't worried about needing to get herself a job for after Christmas. It was all really difficult . . . Was pants . . . Tried to be as realistic as possible without actually saying that it looked like there was a strong possibility that she wouldn't qualify. Was really worried that the kids would pipe up and repeat conversations they have heard me have and drop me in it, but they didn't. She gave me a big hug as she left and said we shouldn't worry, that everything was going to be OK. Felt absolutely awful . . . Racked with sadness.

I am on a late today with a fantastic midwife who I really enjoy working with. She has a way of letting me work independently, but kindly telling me or prompting me to do things if I am confused or miss something. One of the other girls who definitely has a job at my Trust is on her way over. She has an occupational health interview this morning and is popping in for a coffee before she goes. I don't start till 1.30p.m. so have a few hours yet before I have to head out. I have four shifts left as a student . . . OMG! A late today, an early tomorrow, and then Thursday and Friday night (not looking forward to the nights though; the midwife I will be working with isn't so good with students and has that perpetual look of utter contempt on her face when she's talking to me). Then I am done. The next time I go to work it will be as a preceptorship midwife! Aaarrrggghhh! Am so scared!

11.10p.m.

Am drunk . . . very drunk . . . Got to delivery suite today to find a lovely thank you card and a bottle of wine . . . and have drunk half the bottle since getting home an hour ago! Will regret it in the morning when I have to get up at 6a.m. for the early shift, but right now, it feels fantastic! Sooo much has happened in the last few hours . . .

Got to work at 1p.m. and sent a text to student midwife who is possibly about to be discontinued. Was exam board meeting today, and we are all waiting with bated breath to see whether or not we have passed. She replied saying the results hadn't been put online yet. So I suggested she ring them . . . She said that she couldn't get hold of anyone (typical!). I was busy looking after a first time mum who was still establishing in labour after having two Prostins, so I didn't have a chance to look at my phone for another couple of hours (am finding this hard to type 'cos of all the wine! Hee hee hee!!!). Anyway, she got back to me at some point, saying that she'd had a phone call and had been asked to go into uni tomorrow for a meeting. So I asked what was wrong, did she know her results? The reply I got said 'Yes, I failed'. Now, I hadn't had a phone call, so took it that I was OK, but felt gutted for her and asked if she wanted me to go with her tomorrow. She said she was embarrassed enough and congratulations to me. Now I felt really terrible, and offered again to go with her, but this time I got no reply.

Didn't get home till gone 10p.m. but fellow student midwife who I had revised with rang and we talked a lot about what was happening. We have rightly or wrongly concluded that the rest of us are going to pass and that if we had failed, we would have got some sort of contact from the uni today which none of us have. She is going to ring me at work tomorrow to tell me my results, as we are now expecting them to appear online. I need to get 70% or above for my first, but have constant pangs of guilt knowing what student who has failed is going through. Am way too drunk now to comprehend the seriousness of what tomorrow will bring, just have to pray that it will be good news for me (single mother, bills to pay, Christmas presents to pay for . . .). Am going to bed, hope that I sleep and see what tomorrow brings.

Wednesday

Did not want to get up this morning! Felt sick, had a headache, and felt really wobbly . . . perhaps it wasn't such a good idea to drink so much wine last night! Got to delivery suite at 7.20a.m. and had a cup of tea. The woman I had been looking after on my last shift had laboured all night and had needed a forceps delivery this morning. I was allocated her to look after. I did the baby check and the labelling, gave vitamin K, provided her with tea and toast and then left her to rest and spend time with her baby whilst I did all the paperwork. I transferred her across to the postnatal ward a couple of hours later.

Delivery suite was very quiet . . . no-one else came in and we pottered about tidying up and practising suturing on lumps of foam! I kept checking my phone for news of my results but nothing came.

We sat down at about midday to watch a video on the new suturing technique they want us all to use. I had my phone in my pocket and it started buzzing! Was this it? Was this the message I had been waiting for? No! It was a message from one of the girls saying she was going to ring uni because our results weren't online yet. By this point I felt so disillusioned with the whole thing that I didn't have any feelings left at all . . . no anger . . . no disappointment . . . just an emptiness.

Ten minutes later my phone buzzed again. This time the message read 'Just spoken to uni as results not online yet. We have all passed everything except student midwife who had failed summative. The delay was because of that situation. Uni are checking why results not online and will text you when I get them. Congratulations girls x x'. YIPPEE! I have done it! I have passed! I have a midwifery degree! The girls sitting watching the video with me were all looking at me, waiting for my reaction! I read them the message and they all cheered and my mentor came and gave me a big hug and said I was a proper midwife now! Can hardly believe it! Sat there shaking, with a huge smile on my face! I have done it! Bloody hell!

The afternoon girls came on; I was tidying up one of the rooms but was called to take a phone call at the desk. They were all crowded round ready for handover (there was no-one on the board at this point but various messages needed to be relayed). I picked up the phone; it was one of the girls in my group. She knew I couldn't look online for the results, and had promised to ring me when the marks were released. She sounded really sad . . . she said she was really really sorry but that my overall mark was 62%. Fuck. That meant no first for me. Was as if someone had punched me in the stomach . . . I had been so sure that I had done everything I needed to get over 70% in the last trio of essays. Felt absolutely gutted. Everyone was watching and I relayed the news that I had passed, and that I had got a 2:1. They were all so happy for me, and congratulated me, but I felt like I had failed . . .

We stopped for lunch and talked it all through; they were saying that a 2:1 was a bloody good degree and that at the end of the day it didn't matter what mark I had got, but that I was a midwife! I know they are right, but I had so wanted to get a first . . .

As I left that afternoon, I tried ringing the student midwife who had failed. Her voicemail was on and she didn't ring me back till 6p.m. She had gone on her own to this meeting this morning. She had been told that she had failed the postpartum haemorrhage OSCE because her drug doses were wrong. Apparently she had said the same error three different times, and had not corrected herself once. The original markers had failed her, the moderator had failed her, the external moderator had failed her and the board that ratified the results had failed her. Four people had failed her, but she had not been told she was being discontinued! Couldn't believe it when she said that. She had been told that she still had various options! I do feel devastated for her, but there comes a point when enough is enough . . . She had been told that she could appeal against the results (on the basis of lack of support, but she hadn't felt the need to go to the revision sessions!) She could go off sick for three weeks and wait and see whether the board in January passed her (even though four people so far had failed her). She could return to practice for two days and hope that her mentor would give her a level four (as previously she had achieved level three which was a fail). However, she hadn't handed in her portfolio on Monday when she should have done, so that was an automatic fail now too. She still said that she was going to fight it out, and try and do everything she could to get through!

I'm sorry, she still obviously wants to be a midwife, but it just seems like she's grasping at straws and uni are too cowardly to put an end to it all once and for all. Am gutted for her because she is a really good friend. It's all just so sad, and such an awful situation for anyone to be in.

Anyway, I passed I have to try and focus on the positive for me! Got home and sent out a text message to everyone sharing the good news! Changed my status on Facebook to share the news too! Am proud of what I have achieved; still disappointed it's not a first, but then I guess it doesn't really matter. Straightaway I started getting congratulations messages; my mum, nan, dad and father-in-law phoned. Is a wonderful feeling, really hasn't sunk in yet. So, only two more shifts left as a student, Thursday and Friday night. Scary!

Friday

Completely buggered up last night. Had convinced myself that the night shift started at 9.30p.m. so was mooching my way into work at 9.15p.m. (the shift had actually started at 9p.m.) when I met a very surprised-looking preceptorship midwife who, looking quite alarmed, asked me what I was doing there. I told her, and then began questioning myself . . . She didn't believe I had got the times wrong and thought I was joking! But for some really odd reason I cannot explain, I had reverted back to my old shift times as a nurse in a different Trust and was really truly expecting to start at 9.30! Ooops!

Got onto delivery suite and made my apologies to the midwife in charge. Not sure what to make of this midwife, having only worked with her once before; she is difficult to read. Anyway not much going on really . . . I was allocated a thirty-five weeker who was on the way in, possibly in labour. Was told I could do it all on my own so when she arrived. I whisked her to her room and did the initial assessment and popped her onto a CTG. She certainly looked like she was contracting regularly, but they were quite weak. I left her with her hubby and went and bleeped the doc to come and review. He came and did a speculum examination and confirmed that the cervix was closed, and she was not in labour. However, he wanted her to stay on delivery suite until these tightenings had stopped. So, that was my night, popping in and out of the room and checking her CTG. The tightenings finally stopped at 5a.m. and I discontinued the CTG half an hour later. Was disappointed that I hadn't got a catch . . .

Saturday

OMG . . . It's over. I have just woken up after working my last ever shift as a student midwife! Boy, was it a shift! I worked independently (which I am kind of getting used to now, guess I have to get used to it because there is no more signing as a student!). I took over the care of a woman who had just delivered, but had a possible third degree tear. A third degree tear goes right down into the external anal sphincter, and requires a doctor to suture it, so I introduced myself, explained what the plan was and then bleeped the doctor. He came, and confirmed it was what we thought it was. I then had to bleep the anaesthetist and ODA (operating department assistant) and prep my lady for theatre. We transferred her into theatre and I assisted the doctor whilst he sutured. He was a fab doctor and talked me through everything he was doing, pointing out the A&P (anatomy and physiology) at the same time. We came out of theatre and I recovered her.

Went off for my break to find that my first lady had been transferred across to the ward and that three more ladies were on their way in or had arrived already! I was then allocated the care of a first time mum who was contracting irregularly and not coping with the pain. She had already had a VE and was only 2cm dilated . . . the plan was to give her some diamorphine and hope that she settled to sleep. She had the diamorph and was soon away with the fairies; very comfortable, very relaxed and pain-free. I popped in and out just checking on her respirations. I popped my head round the door again; this time it had been about two hours since she had the diamorph. She stirred and told me that she had experienced a long (ten minute) constant abdominal pain and that it was only just going away. I palpated her abdomen and it felt like she was having a strong contraction. Wasn't sure what was going on, she had no abdominal tenderness, and no vaginal loss of any kind, so I popped her onto the CTG for half an hour. Trace was beautiful, baby was a little sleepy (obviously due to the diamorph) and contractions were a little more regular. She had no further constant pains and I checked with senior midwife, who agreed that CTG could be discontinued in the hope she could get some sleep. She did get some sleep! She was still asleep at 8.30 when I made my sleepy way home!

Whilst my lady was sleeping we had a twins lady come in. She was thirty-four weeks gestation and contracting. I wasn't allocated her care, but involved myself by helping the midwife who was. She was a newly-qualified preceptorship midwife and it was her birthday! Anyway, the twins lady began dilating really fast! She was a first time mum – this surprised us all. We transferred her into the bigger delivery room and I got two Resuscitaires, a twins delivery pack, and the Synto infusion for afterwards. By 7a.m. she was pushing and the first twin, a girl, was born within fifteen minutes, and the second, a boy, born fifteen minutes later! It was incredible! I had received the babies and taken them to the Resuscitaires, but they had needed no resuscitation and the paeds were waiting anyhow. Both babies went to SCBU (only because they were thirty-four weekers), and the placenta delivered. As I walked out of the room with the preceptorship midwife we smiled at each other. She was over the moon for delivering twins, on her birthday too! And it was the end of my shift . . . my last shift as a student midwife . . . the last shift where I have the security blanket of being a student . . . Next time I will be doing it for real!

So, I have finished my course and just made it to the magic number forty. I will qualify with forty-one catches to my name. Am disappointed I didn't get any more this week, but being a midwife is about so much more than catching babies as they fly into the world. I have been able to focus on supporting women through labour and honing my clinical skills involving epidurals, augmentation of labour, cannulation etc. so this last week has definitely not been wasted.

My friend on the three-year course, the one who worked as an MCA (maternity care assistant) with me in theatres when I was a staff nurse, is coming over for a takeaway and a bottle of wine tonight! Can't wait to see her and have a good old natter . . . She was such a support to me through my separation, always being there when I needed someone to talk to, so it will be lovely to see her – and get very very very drunk together in celebration that I HAVE DONE IT!

Got my contract through the post today too. And my new Nursing and Midwifery Council (NMC) pin card with my change of name on it! It's official; I have the contract that is offering me the job I have always dreamed of . . . Must have read it through twenty times already, and showed it to the kids, who looked at me with rather bemused faces! Bless them! Starting to panic a bit about the amount of money I have spent on Christmas. Had started off really well-controlled, and now it's kind of gone to pot. I have spent over £100 on the weekly shop for the second week running. Shit, my budget is £40 per week. Am glad I did three weeks of nights last month, which I will get paid for on Monday. And ex-hubby's CSA payments start in January, so that will be a weight off my shoulders. Am trying not to go on about money to the children, but it's hard not to when they keep asking for expensive things every day. Can't help but feel guilty that I can't provide them with the perfect life . . . but then who has the perfect life? Very few people.

Sunday

Had a fun evening with my friend, the second-year student midwife. We got a Chinese delivered and sat chatting and drinking wine, all three bottles of it. Not sure why I haven't got a hangover this morning! She left by 10a.m. and the kids and I got the house ready for a visit from some friends we haven't seen in ages.

Was lovely to catch up with my old friends. Kids have gone to see their dad and so far this afternoon I have removed all the photos of him from around the house, done some washing, bought a lovely wicker basket for my son's Lego and chilled out! Looking forward to my last two days at uni . . .

Week Seventy-eight

Monday

Uni today. Had to drop kids off at sister-in-law's, so made my way into uni on my own. Was glad of the peace and quiet; haven't seen the girls since my disappointing results and really couldn't face it all today – am still so upset, although I know I shouldn't be. Don't know why I can't be happy for what I have achieved, but feel delicate and tearful . . . The student midwife who is almost discontinued wasn't there (she has a sick note for a couple of weeks), so that made things weird too.

Got to uni to find the lecturer who had given me crap marks was teaching us all morning. Great. She is a very 'me me me' person, and after thirty minutes of listening to how wonderful she thought she was I switched off and sat daydreaming. We had a couple of coffee breaks, but I didn't feel that chatty really, and kept myself to myself.

In the afternoon, we got our portfolios back and confirmation from the lecturer that we had all passed. We went through all the pages checking everything and I found a few core skills that hadn't been signed. PANIC! Rang the professional development midwife at the hospital and explained the situation, and she said I should pop to her house this evening and she would sign them for me. I did this, after picking up the kids, and it has all now been signed and I can show it to my lecturer in the morning.

Haven't stopped eating all day and subsequently now feel really sick. Had stopped smoking last Friday (due to my dire financial situ-